50 BEST SHORT HIKES
SAN DIEGO

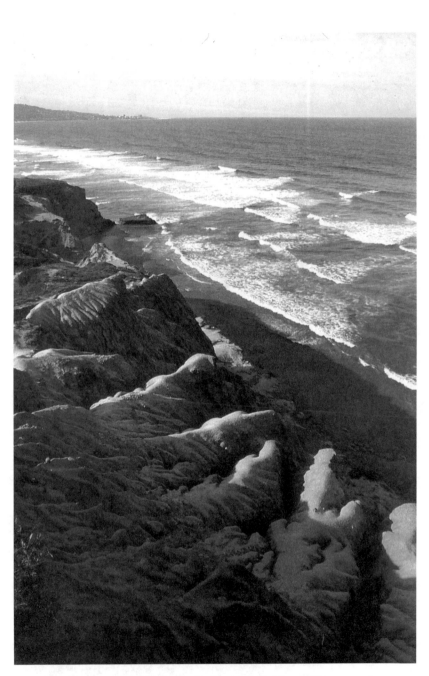

View from Yucca Point at Torrey Pines State Reserve (see hike 19, page 68)

50 BEST SHORT HIKES
SAN DIEGO

Jerry Schad

 WILDERNESS PRESS . . . *on the trail since 1967*

50 Best Short Hikes San Diego

1st EDITION 2011
3rd printing 2016

Copyright © 2011 by Jerry Schad

Front cover photo of Mission Bay at hike 25, Circling Sail Bay, copyright © Stas Volik
Front cover inset photo of hike 9, Del Dios Gorge, by Jerry Schad
Back cover photo of hike 10, Bernardo Mountain, by Jerry Schad
Interior photos, except where noted, by Jerry Schad
Maps and cover design: Scott McGrew
Interior design and layout: Annie Long
Editors: Susan Haynes and Amber Kaye Henderson

Library of Congress Cataloging-in-Publication Data

Schad, Jerry.
    50 best short hikes : San Diego / Jerry Schad.
        p. cm.
    ISBN-13: 978-0-89997-629-7
    ISBN-10: 0-89997-629-8
    1. Hiking—California—San Diego Region—Guidebooks. 2. San Diego
        Region (Calif.)—Guidebooks. I. Title.
    GV199.42.C22S2667 2011
    917.94'985--dc23
                                    2011033166

Manufactured in the United States of America

Published by: **Wilderness Press**
             c/o AdventureKEEN
             2204 First Avenue South, Suite 102
             Birmingham, AL 35233
             (800) 443-7227
             info@wildernesspress.com
             www.wildernesspress.com

Visit our website for a complete listing of our books and for ordering information.

Distributed by Publishers Group West

Safety Notice
Although Keen Communications/Wilderness Press and the author have made every attempt to ensure that the information in this book is accurate at press time, they are not responsible for any loss, damage, injury, or inconvenience that may occur to anyone while using this book. You are responsible for your own safety and health while in the wilderness. The fact that a trail is described in this book does not mean that it will be safe for you. Be aware that trail conditions can change from day to day. Always check local conditions, know your own limitations, and consult a map and compass.

To my wife, Peg Reiter, whose companionship and support during the creation of this book doubled the pleasure of the task of researching and writing it.

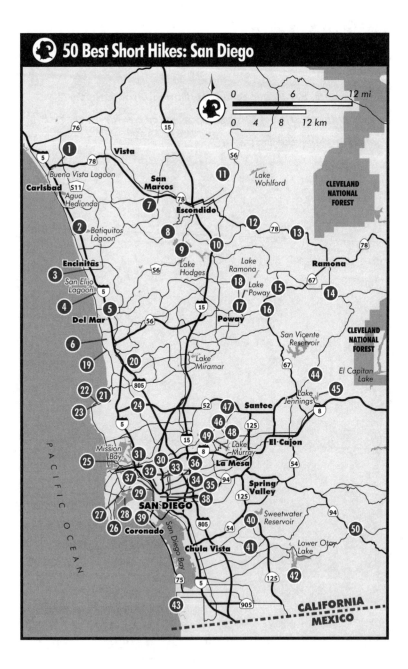

50 Best Short Hikes: San Diego

Contents

Dedication v
Acknowledgments ix
The Very Best Short Hikes x
Introduction 1
Using This Book 4
Map Legend 9

Coastal North County   11

1   Hosp Grove 12
2   Batiquitos Lagoon 15
3   Swami's Beach 17
4   San Elijo Lagoon 20
5   San Dieguito Lagoon 23
6   Del Mar Crest & Beach 25

Inland North County   31

7   Double Peak 32
8   Elfin Forest Recreational Reserve 35
9   Del Dios Gorge 38
10 Bernardo Mountain 41
11 Jack Creek Meadow 44
12 San Diego Zoo Safari Park 47
13 San Pasqual Trails South 50
14 Barnett Ranch Preserve 53
15 Woodson Mountain 56
16 Iron Mountain 59
17 Lake Poway Loop 62
18 Blue Sky Ecological Reserve 64

Coastal & Central San Diego   67

19 Torrey Pines State Reserve 68
20 Los Penasquitos Canyon 72
21 La Jolla Shores 75
22 Coast Walk 78

23   Soledad Mountain 81
24   Marian Bear Memorial Park 84
25   Circling Sail Bay 86
26   Bayside Trail 90
27   La Playa & Point Loma 93
28   Shelter Island 96
29   Harbor Island 99
30   Mission Valley San Diego River Trail . . 102
31   Tecolote Canyon 105
32   Bankers Hill 108
33   Balboa Park's West Mesa 112
34   Balboa Park's Central Mesa 116
35   Balboa Park's East Side 119
36   San Diego Zoo 122
37   The Embarcadero 125
38   Gaslamp Quarter 129
39   Coronado Beach 133

South County   137
40   Sweetwater Trail 138
41   Rice Canyon 141
42   Lower Otay County Park 143
43   Imperial Beach 145

East County   149
44   Louis Stelzer County Park 150
45   Lake Jennings 153
46   Father Junipero Serra Trail 156
47   Oak Canyon 159
48   Cowles Mountain 162
49   Lake Murray 166
50   Hollenbeck Canyon 170

Index   173
About the Author 180

Acknowledgments

50 Best Short Hikes San Diego contains a large amount of adapted and updated material from weekly or monthly columns of mine that have appeared in various publications over the past 30 years. Versions of some of the material are included in my comprehensive guidebook *Afoot & Afield San Diego County*.

Although I have personally researched every hike in this book, I am indebted to scores—too numerous to mention here—of friends, acquaintances, and rangers who have generously provided background information.

I would like to express my appreciation for several individuals at Wilderness Press: Roslyn Bullas revived the *50 Best Short Hikes* concept. Susan Haynes thoroughly and ably edited the text. Scott McGrew and Annie Long handled the book's cartography, design, and layout.

The Very Best Short Hikes

(in alphabetical order)

VERY BEST ARCHITECTURE AND HISTORY

32. Bankers Hill *San Diego's elite residents erected mansions in this exquisitely walkable neighborhood.*

38. Gaslamp Quarter *Stroll among San Diego's most complete collection of historic buildings, now part of the city's liveliest entertainment district.*

VERY BEST BIRD- AND WILDLIFE-WATCHING

4. San Elijo Lagoon *The waterway hosts birds of shoreline and coastal lagoon habitats, as well as small animals.*

43. Imperial Beach *At times, large flocks of seabirds congregate here.*

49. Lake Murray *From hawks and ravens in the sky to egrets and pelicans in the water to coyotes and rabbits on the ground—Lake Murray has it all.*

VERY BEST FOR DOG WALKING

8. Elfin Forest Recreational Reserve *Your pet (if physically fit) can roam in unlimited space.*

17. Lake Poway Loop *Both dogs and their masters/mistresses will enjoy this excellent exercise course.*

49. Lake Murray *The lake's wide shoreline path accommodates all users, including leashed pets.*

VERY BEST FOR EASY STROLLING

22. Coast Walk *Some unpaved trails, but mostly sidewalks, lead the way to La Jolla's best coastal vistas.*

28. Shelter Island *Feast your eyes on the San Diego Bay shoreline as you meander.*

34. Balboa Park's Central Mesa *The paved walk welcomes you into the park's most lavishly landscaped section.*

VERY BEST FOR RUNNING

3. Swami's Beach *Several sets of cliff-edge staircases draw runners for serious interval training.*

25. **Circling Sail Bay** *A near-flat breezy course parallels the Mission Bay shoreline.*

37. **The Embarcadero** *A totally flat course features San Diego's best urban-coastal scenery.*

41. **Rice Canyon** *This mellow course winds down along an unspoiled coastal canyon.*

VERY BEST FOR SMALL CHILDREN

1. **Hosp Grove** *A sun-dappled eucalyptus forest is fun to explore.*

36. **San Diego Zoo** *There is no end to the visual interest and diversions along the way.*

39. **Coronado Beach** *From a small child's perspective, here is where an ocean of sand meets an ocean of seawater.*

VERY BEST SPRINGTIME WILDFLOWERS

18. **Blue Sky Ecological Reserve** *The wildflowers common to inland San Diego County are well represented here.*

19. **Torrey Pines State Reserve** *Coastal-region wildflowers put on a flamboyant show.*

50. **Hollenbeck Canyon** *Wet winters yield early-spring wildflower spectacles.*

VERY BEST VISTAS

16. **Iron Mountain** *The summit vantage encompasses 360 degrees from ocean shore to mountain crest.*

19. **Torrey Pines State Reserve** *The reserve offers the most beautiful melding of land and sea in San Diego County.*

23. **Soledad Mountain** *You'll find superlative urban and coastline vistas.*

26. **Bayside Trail** *Walk this path to spectacular ocean and San Diego Bay panoramas.*

48. **Cowles Mountain** *It features the most comprehensive views of urban and suburban San Diego.*

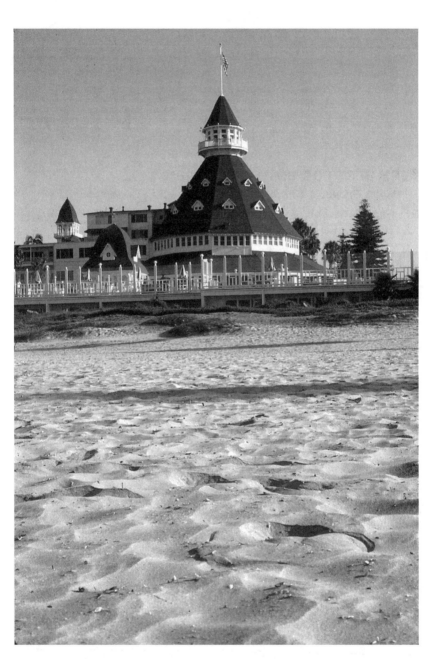

Hotel del Coronado (see hike 39, page 133)

INTRODUCTION

Sunshine. Water and waves. Blue skies and mild temperatures. Sports and leisure. This list of attributes pretty much sums up the image that San Diego projects to the world—and that image is true!

Tourists visiting San Diego for the first time are amazed at the sheer magnitude of park spaces and recreational venues. Everywhere, it seems, people are engaged in outdoor recreation. They're not only swimming, surfing, boating, fishing, picnicking, golfing, and playing tennis but also running, biking, skating, and *walking*.

The focus of *50 Best Short Hikes San Diego* is all about walking, and doing it on the most outstanding 50 trails in this metropolitan region. The selection is so varied that you can match the trail to your time, your mood, your energy level, and even to what shoes you're wearing—or not: The trail surfaces throughout San Diego range from concrete and asphalt to dirt footpaths and sandy beaches.

Geographically, the hike selections include the suburbs and nearby communities that surround the city of San Diego: Just picture the Pacific Ocean coastline from Oceanside in the north to Imperial Beach near the Mexican border. Add to that the various bay and river shorelines. Then color in the hills, canyons, and valleys stretching east up to—within the parameters of this guidebook—about 20 miles inland from the coast. (San Diego County actually extends much farther east than that, encompassing mile-high-plus mountain ranges and a vast desert region. Those remote, eastern areas are covered in detail in a companion book published by Wilderness Press titled *Afoot & Afield San Diego County*.)

The roughly 1,000 square miles of landscape covered in this book offer a year-round mild climate, easy to moderate types of terrain suitable for almost any hiker, and amazingly varied scenery. To put icing on the cake, you may reach the trailheads by car via one of the world's most efficient roadway systems. In the next few paragraphs, let's focus on these superlative claims.

Coastal San Diego County's weather is often tagged as Mediterranean: generally warm and sunny and winter-wet, summer-dry. Despite San Diego's low latitude within the 48 contiguous states, a cool Pacific current moving south along California's coast helps keep the area pleasantly air-conditioned on summer days. Mountain ranges north and east hold cold-air masses at bay during the winter. The bottom line is that daytime coastal temperatures nearly always hover within the 60°F–75°F range. The winter-wet season isn't all that wet: Only about 10 inches of rain fall per year, most coming December–February, and there is no snow! Farther inland, up to 20 miles from the coast for these hiking routes, temperatures aren't quite as mild, with some summer days reaching the 90s, and some winter nights dipping below freezing.

However, where and when heat is a factor, this guidebook coaches you to hike in early mornings or late afternoons—or to save those areas for fall, winter, or spring excursions. And as it is all about day hikes in these pages, you won't have to concern yourself with bundling up in sleeping bags. (Well, a few trails in this book are suggested for enchanting full-moon excursions, but night hiking is recommended only in comfortable weather.)

Another comfort factor is elevation, which is the leading determinant for easy versus difficult trails. While coastal San Diego County isn't highly mountainous, the landscape does rise and fall in a dramatic fashion here and there. As a consequence, the most demanding trails in this book may involve hundreds (but never thousands) of feet of elevation gain and loss—cumulative elevation change—over the course of the hike.

Your payoff for elevation gain in this region is views, views, and views. San Diego is not only highly scenic but also scenically diverse. One route offers a vista of waves and ocean bluffs, while a nearby trail darts into a fragrant eucalyptus grove, and yet another threads through oak woods next to a trickling stream. One trailside panorama encompasses square miles of boulder-frosted mountainsides, while an urban vista frames downtown San Diego's glimmering skyline over the sparkling waters of San Diego Bay.

For a healthy mix of flora and fauna, city and country, you're in the right place when you hike here. The whole of San Diego County (4,200 square miles) is home to more than 2,000 species of native plants and has more biodiversity than any area of comparable size within the continental United States. Some 500 species of birds have been spotted in San Diego County, more than most other counties or parishes in the nation, including Hawaii.

Among the 50 routes covered in this book, you will come upon enough living things to not disappoint. And the hike descriptions tell you what to especially look for among plant and animal species along that trail. Also among these 50 routes, at least a quarter of the hikes weave through some of San Diego's most interesting urban neighborhoods. You'll enjoy the inner city's treasure trove of historical, architectural, and cultural points of interest.

Lastly, from and around the city core, San Diego's freeway system reaches out to nearly every suburb of consequence. That means that parks and open space areas on the suburban fringe are easily accessible. Barring traffic tie-ups on weekday mornings and afternoons, nearly every hike in this book is accessible within an hour or less of driving from the heart of the city.

USING THIS BOOK

The audience for this book is twofold: One is local residents who seek fresh walking routes—or who want to explore their own metro backyards more thoroughly. The other is tourists or business travelers who want a quick post-afternoon-meeting or post-sightseeing bit of exercise.

Whatever made *you* reach for this book, *50 Best Short Hikes San Diego* will entice you to the area's best trails and pathways that are no more than 8 miles in distance and that have no severe elevation gains. Most of the hikes actually fall within the 1- to 4-mile range, which makes them quite suitable for casual hikers.

The most challenging hikes included in this book typically are located inland, rather far from the most densely settled and tourist-friendly sections of San Diego. Such routes may be perfect for half-day-long jaunts, especially on weekends. In some cases, you may have physical limitations to consider. In others, perhaps small children will accompany your walk. Whatever your particular needs or interests, there are hikes for you. Peruse "The Very Best Hikes" section on page x to help you decide where to start.

To select hikes geographically, check the locator map on page iv. It depicts all five regions that are covered in this book and pinpoints the location of each of the 50 numbered hikes. The regional designations—Coastal North County, Inland North County, Coastal & Central San Diego, South County, and East County—are fairly common terms around San Diego. They refer to the metropolitan area of greater San Diego, not to the whole of San Diego County. (The latter includes about 2 million acres of remote mountains and desert that make up the true eastern half of the county, as well as Camp Pendleton, a large Marine Corps base on the county's northern-most coast.) In addition to their position on the overall locator map, the five regions cited earlier each have a map and brief introduction preceding the trail profiles for that area. See page 9 for the map legend.

To select hikes based on elevation, please note that the "Elevation Range" in each hike profile's opening, at-a-glance information refers to the highest and lowest elevation reached on that hike. For hikes involving a substantial amount of *cumulative* elevation gain and loss during the trip—meaning that you'll walk up and down a lot—such ascents and descents are noted in the main hike description.

STAYING SAFE

Every route in this book is safe in the sense that it is a designated public trail or access route, and it is typically popular with other users. Still, you must always be mindful of trail conditions that can change over time and due to weather.

Trails profiled herein vary from dead flat and paved to steep, rutty, and rocky. Please carefully read each trail description before you set out on any of these 50 hikes, and prepare for all of those on uneven surfaces by wearing hiking boots or sturdy walking shoes. If you know that you do not have a good sense of balance, please avoid hikes that could put you at risk of falling.

An example for such caution is the popular route up Cowles Mountain (hike 48, on page 162), the highest point in the city of San Diego. Although there are well over 100,000 separate ascents yearly up the 1.4-mile main trail, the billions of past footsteps on the unpaved path have worn deep grooves into the bedrock of the mountainside, creating an obstacle course of jutting rocks. The danger of tripping and falling isn't such a factor on the ascent, but it is more so on the descent, where stepping down on an uneven surface can result in a fall or a twisted ankle.

In general, you should be as mindful of precautions for these hikes as you are for any trail trekking:

- For all but the very short hikes, wear a lightweight backpack for carrying plenty of water and some snacks. Lack of adequate drinking water can sometimes be a critical issue on any of the hikes located in the hotter, inland areas. It's best to avoid inland hikes anytime the sun is high in the sky during the warmer months of the year. Walking will not be enjoyable at those times anyway.

◘ Your backpack is a good receptacle for extra clothing as well. Because inland San Diego County experiences wider swings in day and night temperatures than coastal areas do, layering your attire is a good idea: Take along two or more middleweight outer garments rather than relying on a single heavy or bulky jacket to keep you comfortable at all times.

◘ Raingear, however, finds only occasional use on the coastal trails of San Diego. Usually, there's plenty of advance warning when a rainstorm is brewing; it is highly unusual for fair weather to turn stormy within a short period of time. But always check the weather forecast.

◘ When the sun is shining (which is most of the time in this region), use sunglasses, wear long-sleeve tops, and apply sunscreen to your

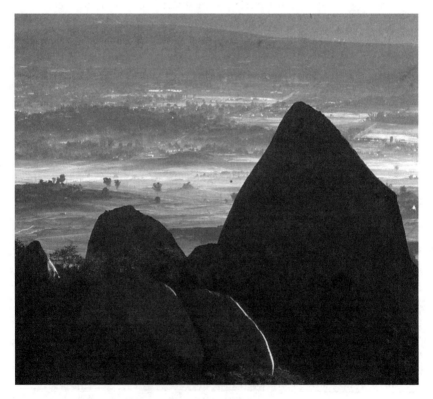

Ramona Valley at Woodson Mountain (see hike 15, page 56)

exposed skin. The higher the sun is in the sky, the more intense the solar ultraviolet. Also, the greater the sun exposure, the greater the danger of dehydration, so fill up those water bottles!

◘ Don't forget to charge up and carry a cell phone before you set out on the walk. Still, do not forget that there are occasional dead zones for cell phone signals once you get away from populated places or well-traveled highways. Thus, as with all hiking, it is wise to let someone know where you are headed and when you expect to return.

◘ Hikers on the more remote trails in this book might want to store a flashlight in their backpacks (if there's any chance of being caught on the trail after dark); a map; a GPS unit, for fun as well as navigation; a whistle (for signaling); and a first-aid kit.

◘ Here and there, especially on trails following the small streams and through oak woodlands, poison-oak growth can be copious. Learn to recognize poison oak's distinctive three-leafed structure, and avoid touching it with skin or clothing. Poison oak loses its leaves during the winter (usually December–March in San Diego), but don't let that catch you unawares. The plant still retains some of the toxic oil in its stems, and it can be extra hazardous in winter because it is harder to identify and avoid.

◘ Rattlesnakes occasionally appear along the nonurban trails featured in this book. Typically, these creatures are as interested in avoiding contact with you as you are with them. But watch carefully where you put your feet, and especially your hands, during the warmer months, as you never want to startle a rattler. Most encounters between rattlesnakes and hikers occur in April and May, when snakes are out and about after a long hibernation period.

◘ Ticks also are an occasional problem, primarily on—again—the nonurban trails. They cling to the branches of shrubbery and wait for any warm-blooded host to wander by. If you can't avoid brushing against vegetation along the trail, be sure to check yourself for ticks frequently. Upon finding a host, a tick will usually crawl upward in search of a protected spot, where it will try to attach itself. If you can be aware of the slightest irritation on your body, you'll usually intercept ticks long before they attempt to latch on.

◘ Mountain lion encounters are possible in the San Diego region, but this situation is extremely rare along the inland-area trails covered in this book. Do, however, keep in mind that you must never run from any predatory animal. Make yourself look large. Do not act fearful. Do anything to convince the animal that you are not its prey.

LEAVE NO TRACE

This guidebook's focus on short hikes within the radius of a major U.S. city does not disregard the importance of preserving the natural environment. Whether you're walking less than a mile through a city park or on an 8-mile backcountry route, please don't overlook your responsibility for your surroundings. Aside from common-sense prohibitions that anyone reading this book likely upholds against littering and vandalism, here are a few pointers:

◘ Never take shortcuts across trail switchbacks. This practice may save you some traveling distance, but it breaks down the trail tread and hastens erosion.

◘ Collecting minerals, plants, animals, and historic or prehistoric artifacts without a special permit is generally prohibited in most jurisdictions. That means common things too, such as pinecones, wildflowers, and lizards. These should be left for all visitors to enjoy—and for the lizards to continue enjoying in their own habitats.

◘ Take note of the signs and information kiosks at the beginning of each walk or hike, and heed all rules and precautions.

Map Legend

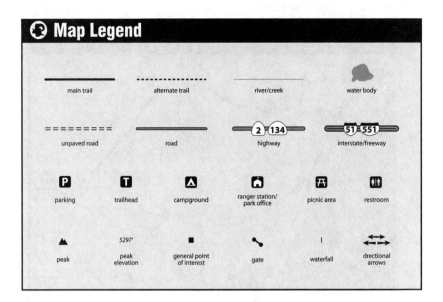

main trail	alternate trail	river/creek	water body
unpaved road	road	highway	interstate/freeway
parking	trailhead	campground	ranger station/park office
		picnic area	restroom
peak	peak elevation	general point of interest	gate
		waterfall	drectional arrows

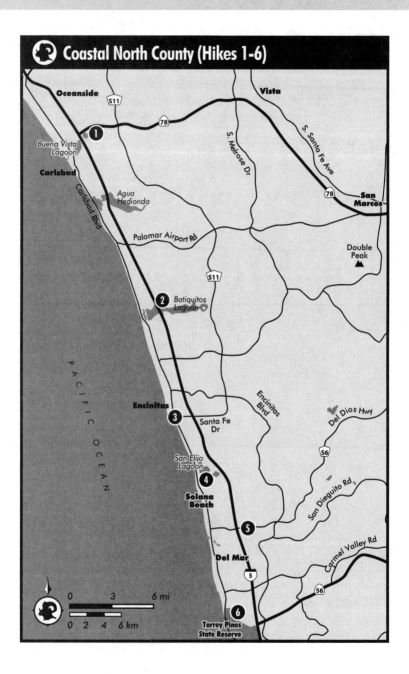

Coastal North County (Hikes 1-6)

Oceanside

Vista

S11

78

S. Melrose Dr

S. Santa Fe Ave

Buena Vista
Lagoon

78

San
Marcos

Carlsbad

Agua
Hedionda

Carlsbad Blvd

Palomar Airport Rd

Double
Peak

S11

Batiquitos
Lagoon

PACIFIC OCEAN

Encinitas

Encinitas
Blvd

Del Dios Hwy

Santa Fe
Dr

S6

San Elijo
Lagoon

San Dieguito Rd

Solana
Beach

Del Mar

Carmel Valley Rd

5

56

0   3   6 mi
0 2 4 6 km

Torrey Pines
State Reserve

COASTAL NORTH COUNTY

Regional Overview

Coastal North County's signature feature is a 20-mile-long, nearly unbroken strand of beaches and shoreline communities. From north to south, they are Oceanside, Carlsbad, Leucadia, Encinitas, Cardiff, Solana Beach, and Del Mar. Compared to the more densely populated core of San Diego to the south, life is a bit slower in these towns. Here, surfing culture has thrived for decades.

But it's not all surfing, all the time. The best hiking opportunities along the North County coastal area center on the immediate coastline, especially along select stretches of sandy beach and also along the margins of several coastal lagoons.

For casual hikers, these venues nearly always offer easy walking and mild—even cool—weather conditions. On the beach itself, there's plenty of surfing talent to ogle, and alongside the lagoons a wide variety of birds will capture your attention.

One caveat: Warm summer weekends may bring throngs of beachgoers to the coastline, making parking a severe challenge. The solution, of course, is to get there early or wait until late afternoon.

◻ ◻ ◻

1 Hosp Grove

Trailhead Location: North Carlsbad, just inland from the coast

Trail Use: Hiking, running, dog walking

Distance & Configuration: 1-mile loop

Elevation Range: From near sea level to 50 feet

Facilities: Water, picnic tables, and restrooms near the trailhead; Plaza Camino Real, a major shopping center, lies 0.5 mile east.

Highlights: Easy hiking, shade-giving eucalyptus trees, and migrating monarch butterflies

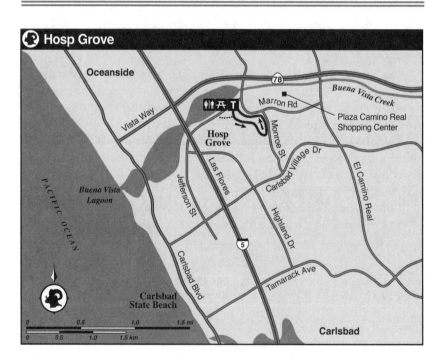

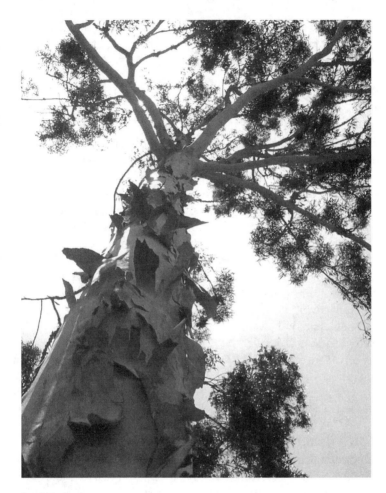

Eucalyptus bark

DESCRIPTION

For better or worse, eucalyptus trees from Australia have become a major component of San Diego County's contemporary urban forest. More than a century ago, entrepreneurs planted tall varieties of eucalyptus all over San Diego County (and in other parts of California) in a misguided effort to produce wood for railroad ties. These trees largely escaped the ax after people discovered that eucalyptus wood cracks and splits too easily for use as lumber. Thus, young and old eucalyptus trees still drape some hillsides just east of I-5 and above Buena Vista Lagoon in Carlsbad, at a place called

Hosp Grove. Within Hosp Grove, the city of Carlsbad maintains a small nature park and trail system, providing a patch of serenity in an otherwise busy corner of North County.

THE ROUTE

You'll find the Hosp Grove Trail rising on the slope behind the park's tot lot. At the top of that short hill, you can swing right (west) toward a dead end, where you can enjoy an eagle's-eye view of Buena Vista Lagoon. This is an especially effective vantage point because you can peer over the tall, obscuring vegetation on the shoreline. Bring along binoculars—or, better yet, a spotting telescope—to observe the birdlife below.

The main Hosp Grove Trail goes left from the top of the short hill, contouring southeast, quite high along a steep slope, through the eucalyptus forest. Not much grows here other than eucalyptus, since the leaf litter from these trees poisons nearly every other type of plant. Eucalyptus branches, though, are attractive to monarch butterflies. This colorful species migrates from summer homes in the Sierra Nevada and the Rocky Mountains, arriving at Hosp Grove and about two dozen other sites around San Diego County in November.

After less than 0.5 mile, the main Hosp Grove Trail descends, turns sharply left, and returns to Hosp Grove Park alongside city streets: first Monroe Street and then Marron Road.

Just east of here, across Monroe Street, additional trails meander amid the eucalyptus trees overlooking the Plaza Camino Real shopping center.

TO THE TRAILHEAD

GPS Coordinates: N33° 10.644121' W117° 20.501883'
Exit I-5 at Las Flores Drive in Carlsbad. Go west on Las Flores a short distance, and then turn right on Jefferson Street. Proceed 0.6 mile to Hosp Grove Park on the right, opposite Buena Vista Lagoon.

2 Batiquitos Lagoon

Trailhead Location: South Carlsbad, just inland from the coast

Trail Use: Hiking, running, dog walking

Distance & Configuration: 2.8-mile out-and-back

Elevation Range: Basically flat, just above sea level

Facilities: Water and restrooms at the start; the nature center at the trailhead is open Monday–Friday, 9 a.m.–12:30 p.m., and Saturday–Sunday, 9 a.m.–3 p.m.

Highlights: Fresh coastal breezes and one of the best bird-watching opportunities in San Diego County. Bring binoculars!

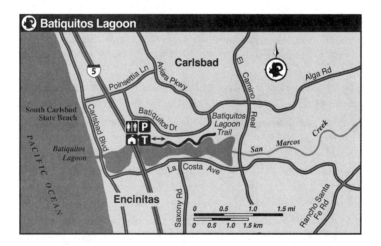

DESCRIPTION

Just beyond the placid north shoreline of Batiquitos Lagoon, white flecks of shell glint in the sunlight where the land begins to rise. Prior to two centuries ago, Native Americans gathered and consumed shellfish here. As generations of natives discarded the shell remains, their middens (refuse piles) grew in size. Keep a sharp eye out, and you will see evidence of those middens today.

The Batiquitos Lagoon of prehistoric and early historic times lived up to its lagoon moniker. Seawater surged in and out on the tides, alternately bathing and uncovering the low-lying, salt-tolerant vegetation. In the 20th century, however, vast loads of soil loosened by agricultural activity and urban development on the lagoon's watersheds were flushed downstream during winter floods. Much of this silt dropped out of suspension near the lagoon's mouth, forming a plug that interfered with normal tidal flows. As a result, Batiquitos Lagoon lost its permanent connection to the ocean and became a stagnating, freshwater lake.

In a giant leap backward, or forward as the case may be, a massive dredging and lagoon restoration project in the 1990s converted the body of water back into a functioning estuary. Millions of cubic yards of sand were dredged from the lagoon's bottom and entrance channel and deposited on nearby beaches or piled up along the lagoon shoreline to provide nesting sites for least terns and western snowy plovers.

Today, you may meander along a delightful trail on the restored lagoon's north shoreline. For the best bird-watching results, arrive here during early morning or late afternoon, when the shorebirds are most active. This also makes a good spot to cool off during one of San Diego's rare summer or autumn heat waves, when temperatures can reach into the 90s.

THE ROUTE

Starting from the Gabbiano Lane Trailhead, head eastward on the main trail. The nearly level pathway curls along the lagoon's north shore, where elaborate interpretive panels have been installed. Traffic noise from I-5, annoying at first, fades as you continue east and pass several small eucalyptus coppices. An iron fence separates a perfectly manicured golf course and upscale housing on your left from the wild assortment of native sage scrub vegetation and nonnative palms, eucalyptus, mustard, and fennel on the shoreline strip you're walking through. (You'll notice along the route that there are four side trails leading north to small parking lots along Batiquitos Drive.)

At a point 1.4 miles from the start, the shoreline trail pulls left and goes under dense eucalyptus foliage. This is a fine resting or picnic spot, and also a good place to turn around and return to the trailhead.

TO THE TRAILHEAD

GPS Coordinates: N33° 5.580840'   W117° 18.018057'

Exit I-5 at Poinsettia Lane in Carlsbad. Proceed east on Poinsettia for 0.3 mile, and turn right on Batiquitos Drive. Continue 0.5 mile, and turn right on Gabbiano Lane, which leads directly to the Batiquitos Lagoon parking lot, nature center, and trailhead.

3 Swami's Beach

Trailhead Location: On Coast Highway 101, just south of downtown Encinitas

Trail Use: Hiking, running

Distance & Configuration: 2.8-mile out-and-back

Elevation Range: From sea level to 100 feet at cliff top

Facilities: Public restrooms and picnic tables at Swami's Park; plenty of beach-flavored eateries on Coast Highway 101, north of K Street

Highlights: Sheer cliffs and well-formed waves; ideal for surfing and beachcombing

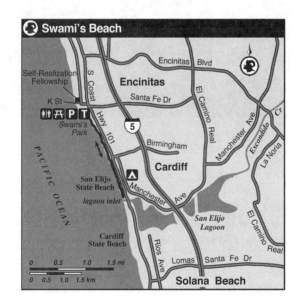

DESCRIPTION

The North County beach vibe finds its best expression in coastal Encinitas, where laid-back surfing and New Age cultures blend. Right below the high perch of the Asian-styled Self-Realization Fellowship (SRF) retreat, called Swami's in deference to founder Paramahansa Yogananda, lies one

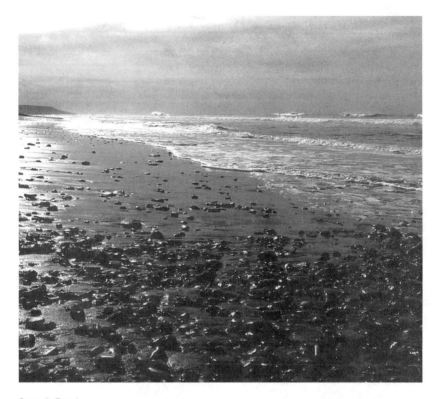

Swami's Beach

of San Diego County's most popular surfing spots. Just take it from the Beach Boys, who referred to Swami's in their 1960s song "Surfin' USA."

Our walk down the beach from Swami's Seacliff Roadside Park, known as Swami's Park and overlooking Swami's Beach, is flat and easy, with no more than a few cobbles here and there to trip you up. If you want, on the way down the beach or on the way back, you can ratchet up the exercise by climbing up and down several staircases. The staircases lead to the cliff-top campgrounds of San Elijo State Beach. These sideways diversions involve little added horizontal distance and plenty of elevation gain and loss if you're game for it.

THE ROUTE

You begin the beach journey at pint-size Swami's Park. From the edge of the cliff, descend the 145 steep steps leading down the sheer slope to Swami's Beach, which is rocky to the north and sandy to the south. Simply head south on the wide or narrow (depending on the tide level) strip of sand that soon becomes a part of San Elijo State Beach. During extreme low-tide episodes in winter, the water level recedes 50–75 yards from the base of the sea bluffs, exposing sandstone reefs rich in marine life. This is less likely to happen in summer or fall because gentle wave action in those seasons tends to deposit a thicker layer of sand on the beach.

Even though the busy Coast Highway 101 lies atop the bluffs, you can't see it. The summertime sensual experience at the water's edge includes the soothing sound of the pounding surf, an ever-steady breeze out of the west caressing your skin, the spicy scent of salt-tinged air, and, of course, sunshine in variable amounts—depending on the cloud cover. (Take off your hiking shoes or sandals and let the lap of foamy water around your feet and ankles enhance this experience.)

As you proceed south, you will pass six separate stairways ascending the bluffs. Likely you'll spot some local runners scooting up and down—or down and up—these stairs for interval training. Some 1.4 miles into the beach walk, you reach the San Elijo Lagoon inlet, where tidal water flows in and out across the beach. This is a good spot to turn around and head back north.

Before you return to your car, or perhaps at another time, consider visiting the SRF meditation garden, overlooking the ocean at the west end of K Street. This serene spot is open to the public at no charge. (See yogananda-srf.org.)

TO THE TRAILHEAD
GPS Coordinates: N33° 2.059257'   W117° 17.526419'
Exit I-5 at Encinitas Boulevard. Go west to South Coast Highway 101, make a left, and travel south past lettered streets (C, D, E, and so on) to K Street on the right. Find a curbside parking space on K Street, or on the west side of 101, or just about anywhere within a reasonable distance of K Street. If you're lucky (fat chance in the summer), you might find a parking space in the small lot at Swami's Park, which is on 101, one long block south of K Street.

4 San Elijo Lagoon

Trailhead Location: Inland from coast between Cardiff and Solana Beach

Trail Use: Hiking, running, dog walking

Distance & Configuration: Up to 4 miles out-and-back if you combine distances on both the East Basin and Rios Avenue trailhead paths

Elevation Range: Sea level to just above sea level

Facilities: No facilities at the main trailheads; access to water and restrooms at the lagoon's nature center on the north shore

Highlights: Five plant communities thrive within a small elevation range; plenty of bird-watching opportunities

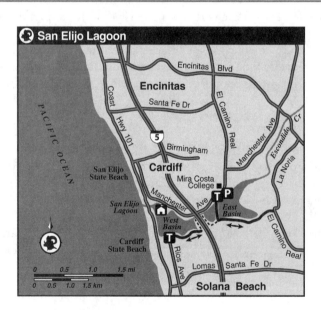

DESCRIPTION

A great blue heron ambles on stilt legs across the reed-fringed shallows, stabbing occasionally at subsurface morsels of food. Nearby, a willowy egret glides in for a perfect landing, scattering concentric ripples across the surface of the lagoon. Both species seem oblivious to binocular-toting humans, who spy on them—from a comfortable distance.

A scene like this is repeated almost daily at San Elijo Lagoon.

West of I-5, in the West Basin part of the lagoon, high tides wash over mudflats and mats of salt-tolerant vegetation. Because of the habitat diversity, you can see a dozen kinds of shorebirds on a typical day. In fact, some 300 bird species have been spotted in and around the lagoon over a period of years, and about 300 species of plants have been identified here.

The East Basin portion of the lagoon, east of I-5, is a freshwater marsh, supported by runoff from Escondido Creek and La Orilla Creek.

THE ROUTE

Two significant hiking routes take you along the shores of San Elijo Lagoon. From the Rios Avenue Trailhead, you can follow beautiful paths that meander along the West Basin's south shore. You will stroll by coastal sage scrub vegetation, which looks bright green in winter and spring and drab in summer and fall. You will also walk through groves of eucalyptus and other nonnative trees. Eroded sandstone bluffs half-hidden behind a screen of vegetation provide an impressive backdrop for the placid lagoon. After about 0.5 mile you are approaching the embankment of I-5, and this is a good place to turn back and return to the Rios Avenue Trailhead.

The second significant hike starts at the lagoon's East Basin Trailhead (east of I-5), opposite MiraCosta College. You begin by following the top of a flood-control dike south to the lagoon's far shore. From there, a trail (with side paths) swings left and traverses the upland part of the basin. One branch leads all the way to La Orilla Creek at El Camino Real, about 1.7 miles from the East Basin Trailhead, and from here you go back the same way.

The accompanying map shows a trail connection between the East and West Basins, but it runs close to busy I-5 and is not inspiring. It is preferable to hike each basin separately from each of their access points.

Note: If you don't have much time, you may want to take the short, looping interpretive trail that originates from the San Elijo Lagoon Nature Center, on Manchester Avenue, 0.5 mile west of I-5. You'll enjoy direct access to the north shore of West Basin. It's the place to go not for exercise, but rather (arguably) for the best chance to see the greatest variety of birds.

TO THE TRAILHEAD

GPS Trailhead Coordinates:
Rios Avenue Trailhead: N33° 0.222723'   W117° 16.334403'
East Basin Trailhead: N33° 0.805922'   W117° 15.594656'
To get to the Rios Avenue Trailhead, exit I-5 at Lomas Santa Fe Drive in Solana Beach. Go west 0.8 mile to Rios Avenue, turn right, and continue 0.8 mile north to the end of Rios Avenue and the Rios Avenue Trailhead.

To get to the East Basin Trailhead, exit I-5 at Manchester Avenue in Encinitas. Go east 0.4 mile on Manchester to the East Basin Trailhead on the right, opposite a satellite campus of MiraCosta College.

5 San Dieguito Lagoon

Trailhead Location: East of the San Diego County Fairgrounds at Del Mar

Trail Use: Hiking, dog walking, running, mountain biking

Distance & Configuration: 2.8-mile out-and-back

Elevation Range: At or very near sea level throughout

Facilities: Trailhead is next to a midsize shopping center with an Albertson's grocery store. Though not built by the publication date of this guide, a visitor center near the trailhead will have water and restrooms.

Highlights: Wide open spaces, fresh ocean breezes, and good bird-watching opportunities

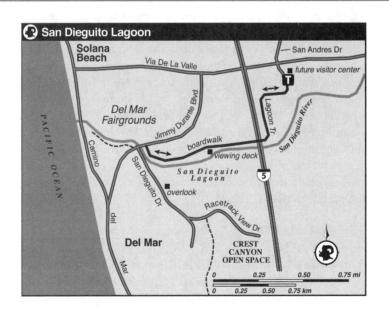

DESCRIPTION

The San Dieguito Lagoon Trail is one of the newest segments in the 55-mile-long Coast to Crest Trail that will eventually stretch from the coast at Del Mar to the mile-high summits of Volcan Mountain near Julian. The Coast to Crest Trail, 25 years in the making, is a part of the fledgling San Dieguito

River Park, whose planners seek to preserve as much as possible the natural features of the San Dieguito River/Santa Ysabel Creek watershed and to provide various means of public access to it. Other sections of the Coast to Crest Trail are featured in hikes 9 and 10 (see pages 38 and 41).

Take along a pair of binoculars if you are interested in bird-watching along the trail. Also, you might pick a hiking time when the tide level is high and the water's edge is closer to the trail. At low tide, the water recedes to a point where it is barely visible from most vantages—and people are not allowed to wander at will into the lagoon and away from the trail.

THE ROUTE

The first 0.7 mile of the trail (for use by hikers and bikers) takes you west toward I-5 and then south to the bank of the San Dieguito River, which at this point flows underneath the concrete bridges of the freeway. As you continue under the freeway and farther west, the white noise of speeding cars mercifully fades, and broad vistas of the lagoon are in view to the south, backed up by the wooded residential areas of Del Mar. At 1.1 miles into the hike, you come upon an observation platform, which marks the start of a planked portion of the trail called The Boardwalk. Bicyclists must turn back at this point; they aren't allowed on the planked section.

The Boardwalk exemplifies 21st-century trail-building techniques, with composite material underfoot and plenty of interpretive panels to educate the public about the cultural and natural history of the lagoon. After about 0.3 mile, you come to the boardwalk's end on Jimmy Durante Boulevard, just south of the Del Mar Fairgrounds. Return the way you came, walking back a total of 1.4 miles.

Note: You could reverse this route and start your walk on The Boardwalk, but good luck with parking!

TO THE TRAILHEAD

GPS Coordinates: N32° 58.830178'   W117° 14.818740'
Exit I-5 at Via de la Valle in Del Mar. Drive east one long block, past the Albertson's-anchored shopping center on the right, to San Andres Drive. Turn right and drive south to the trailhead kiosk.

6 Del Mar Crest & Beach

Trailhead Location: Del Mar

Trail Use: Hiking, running

Distance & Configuration: 4.6-mile loop

Elevation Range: Sea level to 360 feet

Facilities: None at the trailhead; water, restaurants, and small shopping plazas in Del Mar en route within the first 2 miles; water and restrooms at Powerhouse Park and Torrey Pines Beach

Highlights: Pine-dotted canyon vistas and a long stretch of isolated beach

DESCRIPTION

Combining canyon, crest, and sandy strand, this loop hike touches upon every natural landscape that the woodsy community of Del Mar has to offer. The tide-line scenery along the route is some of the best in San Diego County. Be aware, though, that high tides, particularly in winter,

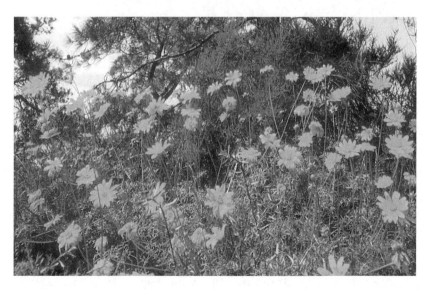

Sea dahlias

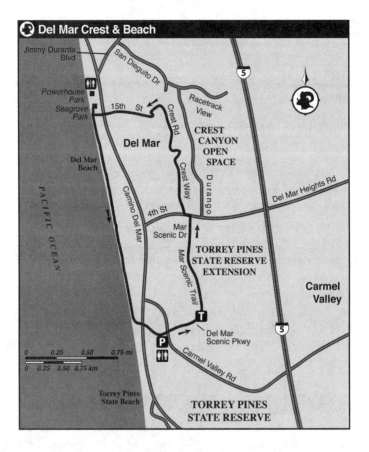

can flood the beach segment of the route. Check tide tables first if you expect to travel along the sand. If the tides do end up flooding the beach, there is a not-as-pleasant alternate route to consider and another choice *not* to consider (see below).

THE ROUTE

Start off at the north end of Del Mar Scenic Parkway, where a sign announces that you are entering the Torrey Pines State Reserve Extension, an annex of the main Torrey Pines State Reserve, which lies south (see hike 19, on page 68). Pets are strictly prohibited in the extension ahead, though the remainder of our route is open to leashed dogs. You'll want to follow the bottom of the ravine on what is signed TRAIL B.

A number of large Torrey pines grace the reserve extension area, their long needles in bundles of five illustrating their identity. The natural range of the Torrey pine, one of the rarest pines in the world, is restricted to the coastal bluffs near Del Mar and to Santa Rosa Island near Santa Barbara. If you want to see more of these beautiful trees, consider a side excursion on the short D.A.R. (Daughters of the American Revolution) Trail, branching to the left of Trail B.

Sticking with the straight-and-narrow Trail B, you arrive after only 0.4 mile at the dead end of Mar Scenic Drive. Keep straight (north) for two blocks, turn left on busy Del Mar Heights Road, and go one short block to reach a traffic signal, 0.7 mile into the hike. Use it to cross Del Mar Heights Road and pick up Crest Way, heading north. Crest Way (signed as CREST ROAD as you continue north) follows the rim of what is called Crest Canyon, a patch of open space on the right harboring picturesque sandstone formations and several large native Torrey pines. Watch for birds of prey wheeling overhead, taking advantage of the thermals.

Crest Road ahead is narrow and without sidewalks. Despite its frequent speed bumps intended to calm traffic, you will need to be vigilant of cars. However, Crest Road traverses one of Del Mar's most exclusive residential neighborhoods, so there's plenty of architectural and floral eye candy to look at. The landscaping includes outsize Torrey pines, which owe their height and girth here to the modern-day miracle of irrigation.

At 1.7 miles into the hike, make a sharp left from Crest Road onto 15th Street. You descend quickly to Camino Del Mar, which is the name of Pacific Coast Highway 101 as it traverses the city of Del Mar. Care for a cup of coffee or other refreshment here? There are lots of choices.

After your break, continue downhill to the adjacent Seagrove and Powerhouse parks (2.2 miles from the start), where you cross the railroad tracks and gain access to the beach. Now go south along the coastline. Low tides are perfect for the 1.6-mile-long, straight stretch of sand-walking that lies ahead. If the beach is flooded by high tide or has unusually heavy surf, you may walk along Camino Del Mar as you continue south.

(*Note:* As another alternative, some walkers and runners will follow the railroad tracks on the bluff overlooking the beach. However, every hour or so, passenger trains whoosh along the rail corridor, often with little warning. Therefore, this guidebook strongly recommends that under no circumstances should you consider this route.)

The stretch of beach below the bluffs is terrific, with the sounds of only a passing train or a happy, barking dog every now and again: This is a popular (and rare) instance of a San Diego–area beach being open to *leashed* dogs year-round.

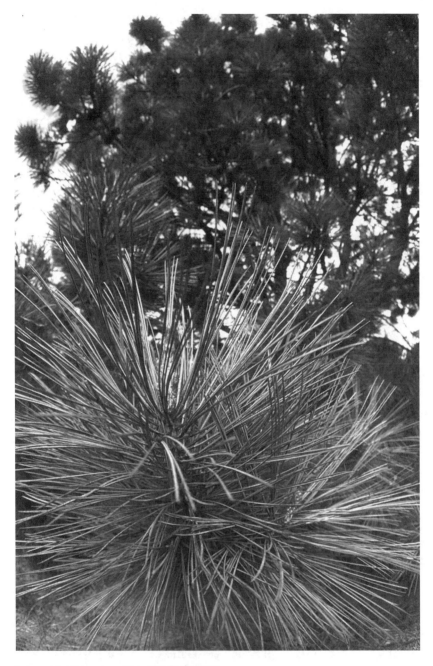

Long needles in bunches of five—it's a Torrey pine!

At 4 miles into the hike, turn inland under the Camino Del Mar Bridge to reach a large parking lot for Torrey Pines State Beach. Walk out to the parking lot entrance on Carmel Valley Road, cross over to the other side, and keep going up the sidewalk of Del Mar Scenic Parkway. Walk all the way to the end of the street, to your parked car.

TO THE TRAILHEAD

GPS Coordinates: N32° 56.300097'   W117° 15.162063'
Exit I-5 at Carmel Valley Road in Del Mar. Drive 1.1 miles west to Del Mar Scenic Parkway on the right. Proceed to the end of that street, where curbside parking is available.

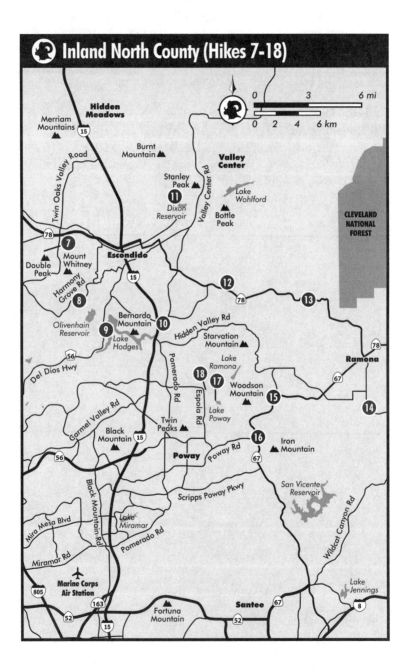

🐏 Inland North County (Hikes 7-18)

Merriam Mountains

Hidden Meadows

15

Burnt Mountain▲

Twin Oaks Valley Road

Stanley Peak▲

Valley Center

Valley Center Rd

Lake Wohlford

11 Dixon Reservoir

Bottle Peak▲

CLEVELAND NATIONAL FOREST

78

7

Escondido

Double Peak▲

Mount Whitney▲

Harmony Grove Rd

8

15

12

78

13

78

Olivenhain Reservoir

9

Bernardo Mountain▲

10

Hidden Valley Rd

Starvation Mountain▲

Lake Hodges

Lake Ramona

Ramona

56

Del Dios Hwy

Pomerado Rd

18 17

Espola Rd

Woodson Mountain▲

67

15

14

Carmel Valley Rd

Black Mountain▲

Twin Peaks▲

Lake Poway

16

Iron ▲ Mountain

56

15

Poway

Poway Rd

67

Black Mountain Rd

Scripps Poway Pkwy

San Vicente Reservoir

Wildcat Canyon Rd

Mira Mesa Blvd

Lake Miramar

Pomerado Rd

Miramar Rd

Lake Jennings

805

✈ **Marine Corps Air Station**

163

52

15

Fortuna ▲ Mountain

Santee

67

52

8

0   3   6 mi

0   2   4   6 km

INLAND NORTH COUNTY

Regional Overview

A wrinkled landscape of rock-ribbed hills, small mountains, and gently sloping valleys characterizes the inland North County region. From such quintessentially suburban communities as San Marcos, Escondido, Rancho Bernardo, and Poway in the west, the land steadily rises eastward toward the even more corrugated interior rural landscape forming the foothills of San Diego County's major massifs—the Palomar, Cuyamaca, and Laguna mountains.

The inland suburban climate is not as benign as that along the coastline. Summer daytime temperatures often rise into the 90s, and wintertime frost occasionally dusts the valleys. Farther inland, in the rural zone around the community of Ramona, summer highs sometimes exceed 100°F. While these temperatures are not remarkably extreme for many parts of the country, it is worth noting that, around here in general, the coming of the sun-splashed summer does not equate to great hiking. It is simply too hot and too dry. Not until October or November do those conditions abate. If you must hike during these potentially scorching months, confine your explorations to early morning or late afternoon and early evening.

When you do hike here, the highly topographical nature of inland North County's landscape ensures that you will be treated to beautiful and often breathtaking vistas. Whether you are cradled in the bottom of a valley or have reached the crest of a peak, the view will almost never disappoint.

Be forewarned that drinking water is scarce along trails that thread through inland North County. The same trails also gain and lose significant amounts of elevation, which only increases the effort of those who hike them. So for reasons of both safety and comfort, hikers are strongly encouraged to take along plenty of water, especially when the weather is warm.

■ ■ ■

7 Double Peak

Trailhead Location: San Marcos, near California State University

Trail Use: Hiking, running, dog walking, mountain biking, horse-back riding

Distance & Configuration: 5-mile out-and-back

Elevation Range: 670 feet at the start to 1,644 feet at the peak

Facilities: Water and restrooms at the start and at Double Peak itself

Highlights: Panoramic views of the entire inland North County area, along with an ocean vista from the top

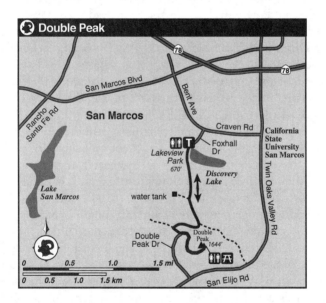

DESCRIPTION

South of the spreading suburbs that cluster along State Route 78, a scruffy ridgeline scrapes the southern sky. Topographic maps note the obscure names of its various high points: Cerro de las Posas, Double Peak, Franks Peak, and Mount Whitney (not *that* Whitney but still the highest of the group). Double Peak, our destination on this hike, is the most hiker-friendly one. Its summit lies within a new city of San Marcos regional and interpretive park that takes full advantage of the peak's panoramic view. Since the park's completion in 2009, it has been possible to drive all the way to the summit from the San Elijo Hills housing development on the south side. Our chosen route, however, goes up Double Peak's mostly undeveloped north slope and capitalizes on a roughly 1,000-foot elevation change. That is appealing, of course, only if you're amenable to a bit of vigorous exercise.

THE ROUTE

You begin at Lakeview Park, next to a small reservoir called Discovery Lake. A flat, 0.8-mile trail, popular with everyone from runners to parents pushing strollers, loops around the lake. Our way to Double Peak, though, takes you across the lake's dam to a paved, traffic-free maintenance road heading south, sharply up a hillside through chaparral vegetation. Soon, you go into and then out of a hillside residential development. Just continue uphill toward a large, hillside water tank. Just shy of the tank, turn left on a fenced dirt path and climb very steeply through chaparral nicely recovering from the last big fire in 1996. North-slope vegetation such as this requires about 40 years of growth to reach a climax stage, and this stand is on its way.

At the next trail intersection (1.2 miles from the start), turn sharply right and continue climbing more moderately until you reach a multiuse recreation path running along the ridgeline. Make a left there (going southeast), and you soon come to Double Peak Drive, which at this point is curling up from the most recently built phase of the San Elijo Hills housing development. Simply get on the sidewalk and continue walking steeply uphill until you reach Double Peak Park's parking lot.

Scattered eucalyptus trees and olive trees, relics from an old homesite, dot the summit itself, and now those trees have been joined by picnic tables thoughtfully placed to frame the spectacular view. The extent of that view depends on the season, with the late fall and winter months generally providing the greatest atmospheric transparency. Even on an average day, you can at least glimpse Southern California's highest mountain ranges (the San Gabriels, San Bernardinos, and San Jacintos) in the north and the shining Pacific Ocean to the west and southwest. On days of exceptional atmospheric clarity, add to that list Santa Catalina Island offshore from Orange and Los Angeles counties and the Coronado Islands off the northern Baja coast. At this point you can retrace your steps back to the trailhead.

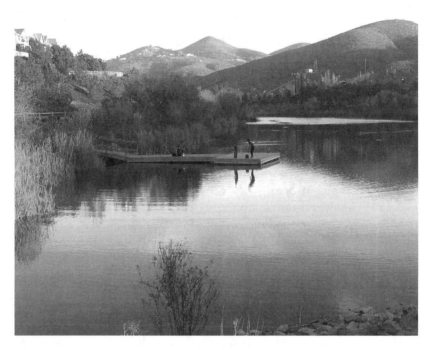

Discovery Lake

TO THE TRAILHEAD

GPS Coordinates: N33° 7.450082'   W117° 10.740960'

Exit SR 78 at Twin Oaks Valley Road (which ultimately becomes San Elijo Road, but you won't go that far) in San Marcos. Turn south and proceed 0.7 mile to Craven Road. Turn right on Craven and continue 0.7 mile to Foxhall Drive. Turn left on Foxhall and proceed to the end of the road and into the parking lot for Lakeview Park and Discovery Lake.

8 Elfin Forest Recreational Reserve

Trailhead Location: East of Escondido, near the community of Elfin Forest

Trail Use: Hiking, mountain biking, dog walking, running, horseback riding

Distance & Configuration: 6.6-mile out-and-back; optional additional 1-mile loop

Elevation Range: 490 feet at the start to 1,300 feet

Facilities: Water and restrooms at the trailhead and at Ridgetop Picnic Area; trailhead also has a small interpretive center

Highlights: Spacious views of inland North County, the ocean, and distant mountains

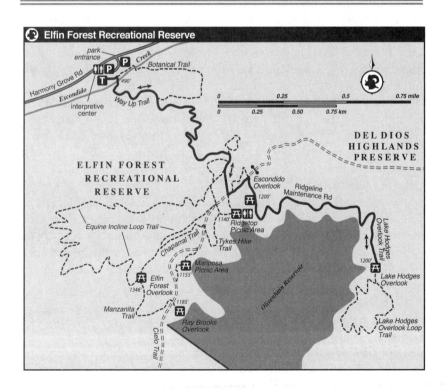

DESCRIPTION

The 750-acre Elfin Forest Recreational Reserve serves two purposes: water management and recreation. The Olivenhain Dam and Reservoir within the reserve holds 8 billion gallons of water, providing an extra, temporary supply for the San Diego region in case an earthquake severs or damages aqueducts that transport water from Northern California. The water-storage scheme also helps to regulate the local demand for electricity. At times of peak electrical energy usage, water released from Olivenhain and falling toward Lake Hodges, below, generates supplemental electricity. During periods of lesser demand, often at night, water in Lake Hodges can be pumped back up the hill to replenish the supply in the reservoir.

The recreational component of Elfin Forest Recreational Reserve and its 11 miles of trails cater to all self-propelled travelers (hikers, runners, equestrians, and mountain bikers) and are uncommonly friendly toward pet owners. At present, on weekdays only, and only at the upper elevations of the reserve, dog owners who have voice control over their pets can let them off leash. *On weekends, dogs must be leashed.*

For small kids, there are short, nearly flat trails near the entrance, where Escondido Creek murmurs and splashes over boulders. The mile-long Botanical Trail, also near the entrance, features interpretive posts keyed to a leaflet. Ambitious hikers and bikers, though, must travel up the hill on the only route—the aptly named Way Up Trail.

They can fashion a number of wide-ranging loops, several miles in length, out of the intricate network of old roads and newer singletrack trails in the upland area south of the reserve's entrance. However, the route described here features the best views of both Olivenhain and Hodges reservoirs. It also offers the most comprehensive vistas of the hills, valleys, and cities near and far.

As this challenging route almost constantly gains and loses elevation, you'll want to start the hike with a full water bottle and replenish it when you reach the Ridgetop Picnic Area on the out-and-back route segments.

Note: Expect to share this and most other routes in the reserve with mountain bikers, as they are welcome and common here.

THE ROUTE

From the reserve parking lot (open at 8 a.m. each day), cross Escondido Creek and begin a crooked ascent on the Way Up Trail. The canyon wall you are climbing is studded with toothlike rock outcrops and dripping with thick, junglelike growths of chaparral. As you may have guessed, the small community of Elfin Forest just west of here and the reserve itself are named after the local chaparral vegetation known as elfin forest. Until late in the spring, this cool, north-facing canyon wall also retains its spring-green grass and exhibits showy clusters of red monkey flower and nightshade.

The Ridgetop Picnic Area, with restrooms and drinking water, comes into view after 1.5 miles and about 700 feet of climbing. You're now on a rolling plateau, and the reservoir lies just ahead. Right before reaching the picnic area, you'll cross the unpaved Ridgeline Maintenance Road. After filling your water bottle, head east (uphill) on that road, and then make a right turn to curl downward past Escondido Overlook (another picnic site). The maintenance road continues east—as do you—along Olivenhain Reservoir's shoreline on a sometimes-uphill, sometimes-downhill course. Your gaze takes in the whole of the reservoir, its surface reflecting whatever color the sky happens to be at that time. On clear, blue-sky mornings, when the reservoir is filled to the brim, the azure surface is reminiscent of an enormous swimming pool with a vanishing edge at the dam on the far side.

At about 2.5 miles into the hike, the road narrows and becomes the Lake Hodges Overlook Trail. You dip sharply to reach the reservoir's shoreline and then climb abruptly back up, eventually reaching Lake Hodges Overlook, with its picnic table and an amazing view of sprawling Lake Hodges below. The Lake Hodges Overlook Loop Trail lies just ahead, and it's worth it to travel the extra 1-mile distance around its looping course. If you do, you get to view the placid waters of Olivenhain Reservoir from different perspectives than before.

Whether you've taken the 1-mile add-on or not, you will begin your return hike from the Lake Hodges Overlook, going back the way you came, negotiating the same ups and downs, only in reverse order.

TO THE TRAILHEAD

GPS Coordinates: N33° 5.193779'   W117° 8.766181'
Exit I-15 at Ninth Avenue in Escondido. Turn west and proceed 0.2 mile. Turn left here, so as to remain on Ninth Avenue. (Auto Park Way continues straight ahead.) Continue 0.6 mile west on Ninth Avenue to a forced left turn onto Hale Avenue. Go 0.3 mile south on Hale, and turn right on Harmony Grove Road. Go 0.3 mile west and turn sharply left to remain on Harmony Grove Road. After another 0.4 mile, you must turn left again to remain on Harmony Grove Road, which becomes a rural byway at this point. Continue for 3 miles to the Elfin Forest Recreational Reserve entrance on the left, near mile marker 6 on Harmony Grove Road.

9 Del Dios Gorge

Trailhead Location: Between Rancho Santa Fe and Escondido

Trail Use: Hiking, mountain biking, dog walking, horseback riding, running

Distance & Configuration: 6.4-mile out-and-back

Elevation Range: 340 feet down to 120 feet (river crossing)

Facilities: Water and restrooms at the trailhead; restaurant across the street

Highlights: The historic Lake Hodges Dam and (rarely) rushing water down the gorge

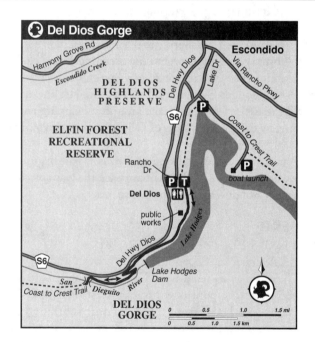

DESCRIPTION

On its roughly 50-mile course from the mountain crest near Julian to the beach at Del Mar, the combined Santa Ysabel Creek/San Dieguito River courses through several steep and narrow canyons. The lowest of these, the

Del Dios Gorge, is partly inundated by Lake Hodges, a reservoir whose concrete-arch dam began to impound the waters of the San Dieguito River in 1918. Below that dam today, a steep section of the gorge remains in evidence. A new section of the Coast to Crest Trail, which will one day stretch the entire length of the San Dieguito River and its main tributary, Santa Ysabel Creek, threads it way right down the gorge.

The best time by far to visit Del Dios Gorge is during winter—better yet if that winter season features above-average rainfall. Every few years, Lake Hodges overflows its spillway, adjacent to the dam. Under the right circumstances, the resulting spray can create a rainbow. Most of the time, because of the dry climate, there's no spillage from the reservoir, and water in the gorge slides gently by or gathers in stagnant pools.

THE ROUTE

From the trailhead, follow the narrow, beaten-down path that swings right, parallel to the shore of Lake Hodges in the direction of the dam. Some mild ups and downs follow, with frequent views of the water below. At one point you pass a large, public works complex on the right. It houses electric pumps and generators that regulate the flow of water between Lake Hodges and the Olivenhain Reservoir, unseen on the high ridge above.

Nearly 2 miles into the hike, you reach a point alongside the nearly century-old, concrete Lake Hodges Dam. Early on, the dam developed troublesome cracks, but by 1937 (following the devastating Long Beach earthquake of 1933) the dam had been strongly reinforced. Other than some painted-over graffiti, the dam retains its old-world architectural charm.

Just beyond the dam, the trail pulls right alongside Del Dios Highway. Soon, you turn abruptly left and descend toward the bottom of the gorge on an unpaved service road, doubling as the trail route. Notice the remnants of a flume that formerly connected Lake Hodges to a smaller storage facility, San Dieguito Reservoir, some 4 miles away.

As you continue downhill and downstream, there's never a point where the noise from nearby Del Dios Highway isn't apparent, but at least you can admire the steeply rising far wall of the gorge and the scattered willows, oaks, and granite outcrops down along the riverbed. Restoration efforts are under way, which will ultimately improve the habitat alongside the river, encourage the growth of native vegetation, and provide better foraging and nesting for birds.

At 3.2 miles from the start, the trail swings sharply left and crosses the San Dieguito River on an elaborate iron footbridge. Further travel on the trail-in-progress ahead will someday allow you to walk all the way

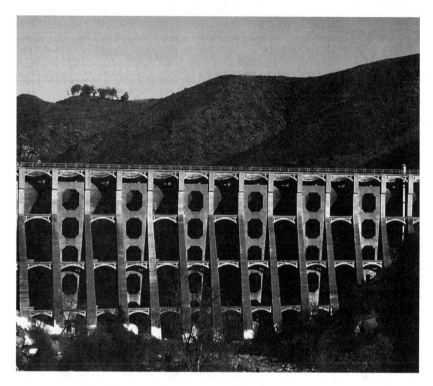
Lake Hodges Dam

out to the beach at Del Mar, but our hike ends here at the bridge. Return the same way you came.

TO THE TRAILHEAD
GPS Coordinates: N33° 3.776100'   W117° 7.181396'
Exit I-15 at Via Rancho Parkway. Drive west on Via Rancho for 3.5 miles, turn left at the Del Dios Highway traffic light, go 2 miles farther to Rancho Drive (traffic light), and turn left again. Rancho Drive goes downhill for 0.3 mile to a San Dieguito River Park trailhead and staging area on the right. The famed Hernandez Hideaway biker bar restaurant lies across the street from the trailhead.

10 Bernardo Mountain

Trailhead Location: South Escondido

Trail Use: Hiking, running, mountain biking, dog walking

Distance & Configuration: 7.2-mile out-and-back

Elevation Range: 330 feet at the start to 1,150 feet at the summit

Facilities: Water and restrooms at the trailhead; myriad facilities at the giant North County Fair shopping center, 0.5 mile north of the trailhead

Highlights: A summit view encompassing the Lake Hodges reservoir, plus valleys and mountains as far as the eye can see

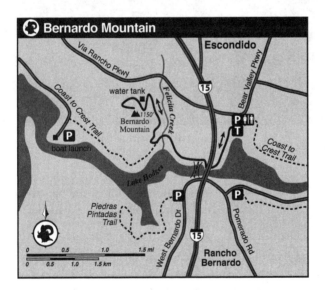

DESCRIPTION

The massive bulk of Bernardo Mountain rises from the north shoreline of Lake Hodges, almost like a smooth-sided pyramid. The summit area of the mountain was purchased for inclusion in the San Dieguito River Park in 2002, and that gave public access for hikers and bikers. The park, designed to preserve as much of nature as possible within the San

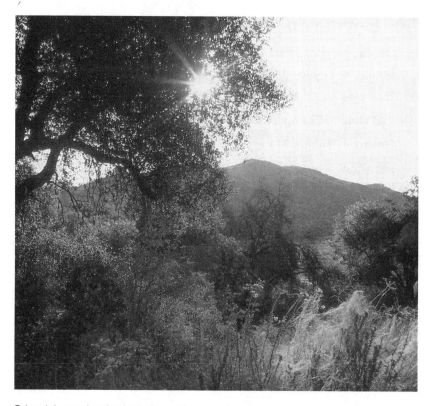

Oak and chaparral on the shore of Lake Hodges

Dieguito River/Santa Ysabel Creek watershed, stretches about 50 miles between the coastline at Del Mar and Volcan Mountain near Julian.

THE ROUTE

Start off from the Sunset Drive Trailhead by heading south, parallel to I-15, initially on a wide, concrete walkway. After about 0.4 mile, the pathway turns sharply right and passes under the freeway bridge that goes over the east arm of Lake Hodges. You'll soon hook up with a dirt trail following the lake's north shoreline, going west. A short distance later, you'll come to the north end of an elaborate footbridge, completed in 2009, that spans the lake and runs parallel to the freeway. If you want to make a short, optional side trip, cross the bridge and then return to this route.

At 1.6 miles into your trip, you cross Felicita Creek, a small perennial brook deeply shaded by oaks, sycamores, palms, and other water-loving vegetation. After the creek crossing, make a right on the first available singletrack trail, heading north toward Bernardo's summit.

You ascend gradually at first through scrubby chaparral vegetation, with the oaks and sycamores of Felicita Creek just below you on the right and Bernardo Mountain rising on the left. By about 2.5 miles, you've swung around to the north side of the mountain, where the views become more expansive. Much of what comes into view in the north are rural housing areas surrounding the city of Escondido. Stay left (uphill) at the next two trail intersections, always heading upward.

You continue ascending or contouring in a zigzag pattern, passing a large water tank at 3.2 miles and finally reaching the rocky summit at 3.6 miles. From this noble vantage point, you can clearly visualize the patchwork of urban, suburban, and wildland that inland North County has become. The white noise of traffic on I-15 wafts upward to you—but peering in certain other directions, you see little apparent human impact on the landscape. Westward, down the valley below Lake Hodges, a slice of Pacific Ocean is visible on clear days.

When you're ready to go, return the way you came.

TO THE TRAILHEAD

GPS Coordinates: N33° 4.038599'   W117° 3.875399'
Exit I-15 at Via Rancho Parkway in south Escondido. Go east one long block to Sunset Drive. Turn right and drive 0.2 mile to the San Dieguito River Park trailhead and parking area.

11 Jack Creek Meadow

Trailhead Location: North Escondido

Trail Use: Hiking, mountain biking, running, dog walking

Distance & Configuration: 5.6-mile loop

Elevation Range: 1,170 feet to 1,460 feet

Facilities: Water, restrooms, picnic grounds, and campgrounds in the Dixon Lake Recreation Area, near the trailhead

Highlights: Serene scenery, ranging from grassy meadow to oak woodland, nearly all of it in its natural state

DESCRIPTION

Daley Ranch preserve, a former working ranch that passed into public ownership in the 1990s, occupies the only large undeveloped acreage in the city of Escondido. Here, we spotlight the best introductory hike Daley Ranch offers, taking you to a remote elevated valley that is completely removed from sight and sound of civilization.

The hike or bike ride to Jack Creek Meadow is outstanding when taken during the cooler months, and it's tolerably comfortable on most summer days, assuming you travel in the early morning or late afternoon. If you live or work in inland North County, consider this route for a bit of quick and intense exercise: a speed walk of perhaps 90 minutes, a 60-minute jog, or a 40-minute mountain-bike ride.

THE ROUTE

At the Daley Ranch parking lot and staging area, step around the Daley Ranch gate and walk uphill, rather steeply, on the paved access road ahead. This service road, named Ranch House Trail, reaches a summit at 0.4 mile and then starts descending into live-oak woods. On the right, you get a glimpse of the largest of several old stock ponds on the ranch, its shoreline guarded by tall cattails.

After 1.2 miles, pavement on Ranch House Trail ends and the quaint redwood Daley ranch house (generally closed to public visitation) sits to the left. Descendants of Robert Daley, who settled in this valley in 1869, erected the house in 1928. Continue north another 200 yards past

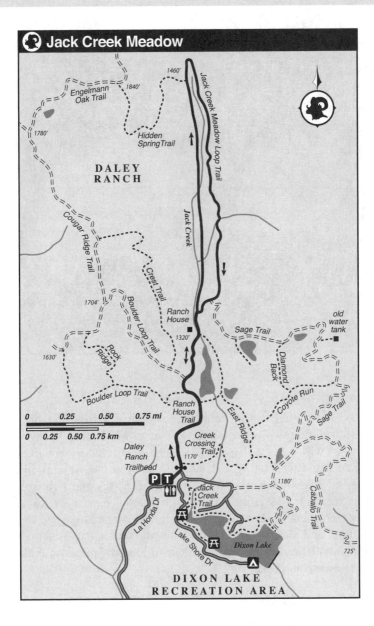

Jack Creek Meadow

various outbuildings to the beginning of the dirt-road route signed JACK CREEK MEADOW.

The elongated loop you follow—Jack Creek Meadow Loop Trail—takes you around the margins of a linear meadow, so narrow and so straight that

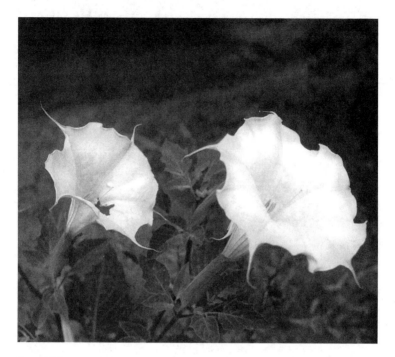

Sacred datura

it suggests some underlying, probably ancient fault structure. The meadow, lined with a dark-green row of coast live oaks and backed up by steep slopes shaggy with mature chaparral, looks impressive when seen in early-morning or late-afternoon light. Close at hand you pass several gnarled specimens of Engelmann oak, with gray-green leaves and light-colored bark. The meadow grasses are almost entirely nonnative, typically of an emerald-green color for about 3 months in the winter and bleached yellow-brown after 1 or 2 months of springtime sun and prolonged drought.

After completing the inspirational loop around the meadow, return to your car the way you came.

TO THE TRAILHEAD

GPS Coordinates: N33° 10.008302'   W117° 3.118737'

Exit I-15 at El Norte Parkway in north Escondido. Drive 3 miles east and make a left turn (north) on La Honda Drive. Drive 1 mile uphill to the end of the road, where you will find the large parking lot and staging area for Daley Ranch on the left, just short of the Dixon Lake entrance.

12 San Diego Zoo Safari Park

Trailhead Location: Just east of Escondido

Trail Use: Hiking

Distance & Configuration: 3.5-mile loop, including two spurs

Elevation Range: 400 feet to 700 feet

Facilities: Water, restrooms, and snack bars along much of the route

Highlights: Native and nonnative flora and fauna from around the world

DESCRIPTION

The San Diego Zoo Safari Park (formerly San Diego Zoo's Wild Animal Park) sprawls over an 1,800-acre expanse chosen for its resemblance to Africa's most productive wildlife areas. Make no mistake—virtually everything here is artificial. That doesn't diminish in the least the park's goal of preserving rare species of plants from around the world and rare animals, particularly those of the African savannas. More than four decades worth of landscape improvements have rendered this less of a zoo and more of a safari experience, as the park's title expresses.

Parking and admission fees are high, but you can mitigate them by joining the Zoological Society of San Diego. The society operates the San Diego Zoo in Balboa Park as well as the Zoo Safari Park. Repeated free visits to both facilities then become possible during a year's membership.

This is one zoo, perhaps like no other, where a walkabout resembles a true hike, albeit one where a good fraction of the scenery is engineered. Of many possible routes, the one described below, circling the perimeter of the park, is navigationally the easiest and offers you the greatest variety of sights. Including two spurs near the end of the loop, the route covers 3.5 miles altogether. It also avoids almost entirely the heavily trafficked footpaths, so you can actually get some heart-pounding exercise if you choose not to linger at the exhibits along the way. Do pick up a detailed map (free with admission) at the park's entrance.

THE ROUTE

From the entrance, stay to the right, first entering and later exiting the Wings of the World aviary. Ahead, just stick with the navigational rule

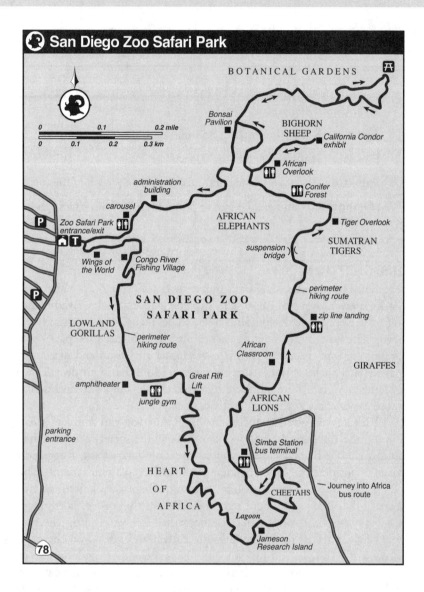

San Diego Zoo Safari Park

BOTANICAL GARDENS

Bonsai
Pavilion

BIGHORN
SHEEP

California Condor
exhibit

African
Overlook

Conifer
Forest

administration
building

carousel

Zoo Safari Park
entrance/exit

AFRICAN
ELEPHANTS

Tiger Overlook

SUMATRAN
TIGERS

Wings of
the World

Congo River
Fishing Village

suspension
bridge

perimeter
hiking route

SAN DIEGO ZOO
SAFARI PARK

zip line landing

LOWLAND
GORILLAS

perimeter
hiking route

African
Classroom

GIRAFFES

amphitheater

jungle gym

Great Rift
Lift

AFRICAN
LIONS

parking
entrance

Simba Station
bus terminal

HEART

OF

AFRICA

CHEETAHS

Journey into Africa
bus route

Lagoon

Jameson
Research Island

78

0   0.1   0.2 mile
0   0.1   0.2   0.3 km

that you always swing to the right, except at paths that dead-end quickly or on paths and roads posted NO ENTRY.

You'll pass through the Congo River Fishing Village (with its faux stream), the lowland gorilla exhibit, and eventually arrive at the Great Rift Lift, the launching platform for a tethered passenger balloon. Check out the view from there, which replicates an African savanna spread in the distance. Take the stairs from there down to the Heart of Africa entrance, where you pick up a meandering path, paved and wood-planked, down past numerous animal and bird exhibits and over an artificial lagoon.

On the far side of the lagoon, the path climbs upward past the cheetah zone, the Journey into Africa bus-tour terminal, and the lion exhibit. As ever, swing right at every junction. Once past the lions, you'll be traversing paved and unpaved paths in the backcountry zone of the park that closes before sunset year-round. It is here that you will likely spot at close range wild mule deer from the surrounding area that seem to enjoy taking advantage of the unenclosed habitat of the park.

Proceed north past the zip line landing spot, lurch over a rocking suspension footbridge, pass the Tiger Overlook, and enter a deeply shaded zone of densely spaced conifers from around the world. As you continue making rights, the turns will eventually take you east to see desert bighorn sheep and a California condor exhibit. You will also enjoy a terrific view of the savanna below and the distant San Pasqual Valley.

Turn back from the condor exhibit area and return to the main looping route. In a short while, near the Bonsai Pavilion, you pick up a service road to the right and are directed by signage to a trail leading to the Baja botanical gardens, up along a gentle hillside, your second side trip.

Magnificent desert succulents thrive here for sure, but that's not all. You also will see native sage scrub, chaparral, and riparian vegetation, and most specimens are meticulously identified. You must explore all looping side paths to see everything.

Early or late in the day, the Zoo Safari Park landscape and its background skyline of rocky peaks look especially beautiful from here. At one spot, a picnic table under a shade ramada fringed with palm fronds invites you to sit and contemplate the scene.

From this serene and seldom-visited retreat, go back to the main looping route and return down through the visitor-clogged park spaces to the entrance and exit gates, where you started.

TO THE TRAILHEAD

GPS Coordinates: N33° 5.991004'   W117° 0.059938'
Exit I-15 at Via Rancho Parkway in south Escondido. Proceed east on Via Rancho Parkway 1 mile to San Pasqual Road. Turn right, continue 3 miles, and turn right (east) on State Route 78. Go 1 mile farther to the Zoo Safari Park on the left.

13 San Pasqual Trails South

Trailhead Location: Between Escondido and Ramona in north-central San Diego County

Trail Use: Hiking, running, dog walking

Distance & Configuration: 7.2-mile out-and-back (including two spurs)

Elevation Range: 680 feet at the start to 1,755 feet at the highest summit

Facilities: None near the trailhead; water and restrooms at San Pasqual Battlefield State Historic Park (if open), 4 miles west

Highlights: Spacious views of mountains, valleys, and the distant Pacific coastline

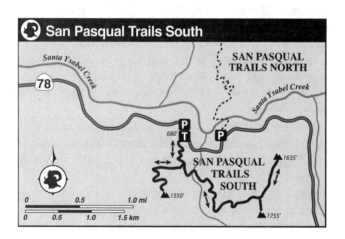

DESCRIPTION

The San Dieguito River Park's San Pasqual (also known as Clevenger Canyon) trail system lies within San Diego County's arid interior, east of Escondido. These trails expose you to steep, boulder-frosted hillsides, clothed in a tough mixture of vegetation that is recovering from the 2007 Guejito Fire. You will see fast-growing sage scrub plants and slower-growing chaparral. Because of the high summer temperatures, it's best to hike in cool months. Here and there you'll benefit from the shade of coast live oak trees—hardy survivors that have seen many wildfires over a span of decades or longer.

The trail system consists of two networks, north and south of State Route 78, but here we'll focus on the south trail system, which has been better maintained since the fire.

THE ROUTE

The complete reconnaissance of the south-side trails involves a 7.2-mile round trip. While the elevation ranges 680–1,755 feet, you will experience a *cumulative* elevation gain of 1,900 feet and loss of 1,900 feet. It's worth it: If you go on an unusually clear day, the coast-to-mountain views on the high points reached via these trails can be truly stunning.

Start your walk from the trailhead by zigzagging uphill 0.5 mile to the first marked trail junction. Choose the right branch (west) for a

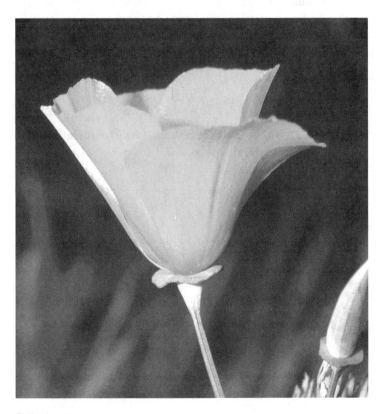

California poppy

relatively easy climb to a 1,550-foot knoll. From this vantage point, you can spot the blue or silvery (depending on the time of day) ocean surface on clear winter days.

Return the same way, and when you are back at the trail intersection, head up the more challenging east branch. You begin with a short passage through a spooky ravine, replete with a tangle of live-oak limbs, wild-cucumber and poison-oak vines, and a mantle of mosses. On the far side, you tackle switchback segments of trail leading toward a prominent, monolithic boulder on a high ridge to the east. After passing within a few yards of the boulder, there's a side trail on the right leading to a 1,755-foot viewpoint—good for another view to the west. Return to the main east branch trail and continue toward a 1,635-foot bump on a ridge 0.5 mile northeast. That's where, on a clear day, you get a stupendous view of upper San Pasqual Valley, a slice of ocean horizon in the west, and the distant, blue-tinted mountains in the east. Almost straight down 1,000 feet, you can spy cars, which appear toylike as they make their way along the sinuous asphalt ribbon of SR 78. Return to the trailhead along the main trail, bypassing your earlier side trips.

TO THE TRAILHEAD

GPS Coordinates: N33° 5.108163'   W116° 55.333557'
From any major I-15 exit in Escondido, follow signs to the San Diego Zoo Safari Park, on SR 78 east of Escondido (see page 49 for details). The San Pasqual South Trailhead is located 5.3 miles east of the Safari Park entrance, on the right (south) side of SR 78.

14 Barnett Ranch Preserve

Trailhead Location: South of Ramona, in north-central San Diego County

Trail Use: Hiking, horseback riding, dog walking, mountain biking, running

Distance & Configuration: 5.4-mile out-and-back (including two spurs)

Elevation Range: 1,400–1,500 feet

Facilities: A couple of picnic tables along the route; all other services in Ramona, 3 miles north

Highlights: Rolling grasslands reminiscent of Montana's Big Sky Country

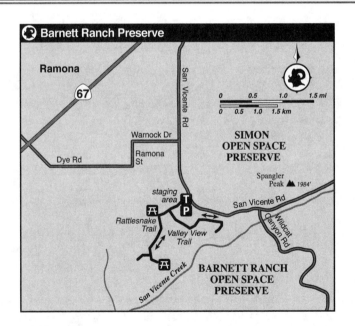

DESCRIPTION

Barnett Ranch Open Space Preserve, operated by the county of San Diego, is one of several former cattle ranches newly converted to parkland throughout San Diego's suburban and rural areas. An ongoing project called the Multiple

Species Conservation Program aims to protect key parcels such as this one for the benefit of indigenous flora and fauna, as well as for human visitors.

Barnett Ranch Open Space Preserve spreads across about 728 acres of gently rolling grasslands and sage- and chaparral-covered slopes. The preserve offers multiuse trails (former unpaved ranch roads) that take you to nearly every corner of the property.

THE ROUTE

From the Barnett Ranch staging area, this outing includes two out-and-back multiuse routes: the Rattlesnake Trail and the Valley View Trail. The Rattlesnake Trail is terrific, once you get beyond the initial 0.5-mile dirt path alongside a rural driveway. You will curve into a sensuously rounded vale, cross a freshwater marsh with verdant grasses and swaying cattails

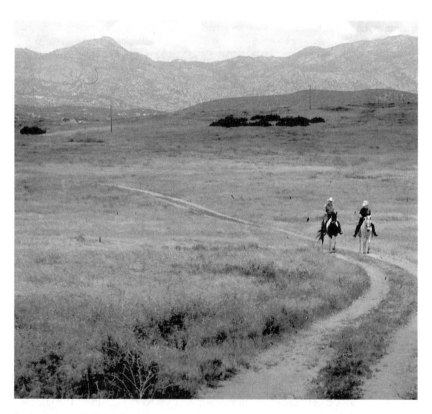

Equestrians on the Valley View Trail

(and a nearby picnic table), and climb a bit more to a second picnic table next to some oaks singed by the 2003 Cedar Fire.

In the spring—March or April following a wet winter—the landscape looks as green as Ireland, and wildflowers are popping up everywhere. On a summer visit, you'll likely spot ravens and hawks gliding on thermals. Under the warm sun, mini-vortexes of heated air might carve raspy-sounding grooves through the dry grasses, like ghosts dancing.

On the way back, the Valley View Trail, which branches east from Rattlesnake Trail, seems inferior, as its destination is a pair of vantage points also occupied by steel pylons supporting a high-voltage power line. You do get a view, though, of San Vicente Creek's valley below, which is not-so-picturesquely dotted with various dwellings and ranching infrastructure. Return the way you came, and take a right at the intersection with Rattlesnake Trail to arrive back at the trailhead.

TO THE TRAILHEAD
GPS Coordinates: N33° 0.035219'   W116° 51.876540'
From the junction of State Route 67 and State Route 78 in the center of Ramona, turn south on Tenth Street. Within four blocks, Tenth Street becomes San Vicente Road. Continue a total of 3 miles to Deviney Lane on the right (west) side of San Vicente Road. The well-marked trailhead and equestrian staging area for Barnett Ranch lies here. For some travelers, a shortcut to San Vicente Road from SR 67 via Dye Road, Ramona Street, and Warnock Drive might save time.

15 Woodson Mountain

Trailhead Location: Between Poway and Ramona, in north-central San Diego County

Trail Use: Hiking, dog walking, running, biking, night hiking

Distance & Configuration: 3.6-mile out-and-back

Elevation Change: 1,680 feet at the start to 2,894 feet at the summit

Facilities: No facilities nearby other than in Ramona or Poway, each several miles away

Highlights: Outsize boulders pepper the slopes of this wild-looking mountain. Topside views are some of the broadest in San Diego County.

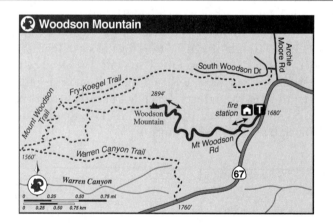

DESCRIPTION

Native Americans called it Mountain of Moonlit Rocks, an appropriate name for a landmark visible, even at night, from great distances. Later settlers dubbed it Cobbleback Peak, a name utterly descriptive of its rugged, boulder-strewn slopes. But for more than a century, the peak has appeared on maps simply as Woodson Mountain, after Confederate dentist Dr. Marshall Clay Woodson, who homesteaded at its foot in 1895. Today, Woodson Mountain is a local landmark, renowned among rock climbers all over Southern California as well as among local hikers, who are able to ascend the peak from a variety of directions.

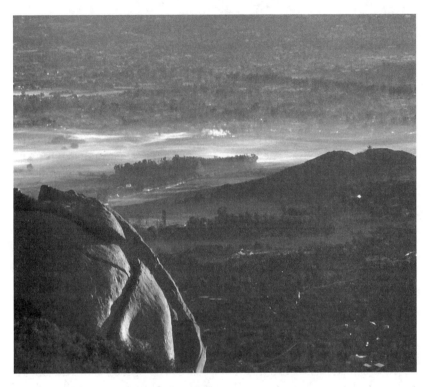

Ramona Grasslands as seen from Woodson Summit area

The eastern approach described here uses a paved service road closed to motor traffic. Although very steep in places, the smooth-surfaced pathway lends itself well to after-dark hiking, provided you have a flashlight. The route is also suitable for road and mountain biking, but that's practical only if your bicycle has extremely low gears and the brakes are in tip-top shape.

Summer days are typically too hot for climbing Woodson. Early morning or late afternoon sometimes works spectacularly, though. At those times, during much of the warmer half of the year, stratus clouds cover the coastal landscape up to an elevation of 1,000–2,000 feet. Woodson's 2,894-foot summit often pokes above that dense blanket of cottony clouds, much to the pleasure of early-morning visitors. Incredible sunset views often reward late-afternoon or evening hikes, and that advantage is doubled whenever there's a full moon. With every full moon on a clear evening, you can witness a near-simultaneous sunset in the west and moonrise in the east.

THE ROUTE

A small sign marks the trailhead at the entrance to the fire station. From that starting point, follow a narrow path south though some oak trees alongside State Route 67. Within only 0.1 mile, you arrive at the paved service road. Turn right and chug 1.5 miles up, up, and up to Woodson's antenna-topped summit, some 1,200 feet higher than your starting point. Everywhere you look there are rounded boulders galore. The beige and light-gray rocks of Woodson Mountain and several of its neighboring peaks are of a type that geologists call Woodson Mountain granodiorite. When exposed at the surface, they weather into huge spherical or ellipsoidal boulders with smooth surfaces. The largest of them have a tendency to cleave apart along remarkably flat planes, leaving gaps of several inches to several feet. Sometimes, half of a split boulder will roll away, leaving a vertical and almost seamless face behind. Near the top of the mountain, you'll feel absolutely dwarfed as you pass between boulders the size of large houses.

As you approach the summit, the incline moderates somewhat, and you can catch your breath. On the summit itself you'll have to move around a bit, dodging antenna installations, for views in every direction. To enjoy the optimum western view, walk about 0.2 mile farther west and downhill from the summit, along the narrow summit ridge. After passing several antenna towers, you'll reach a vantage point overlooking Poway and much of the north county, not to mention a vast sweep of the Pacific Ocean—if the atmosphere is clear enough. Very near that spot, don't miss the sight of an amazing cantilevered "potato-chip" flake of rock, the result of exfoliation and weathering of a huge boulder.

When it's time to leave, head back the same way you came. The traction on the paved road is excellent, but it's a real knee banger due to the steep slope.

TO THE TRAILHEAD

GPS Coordinates: N33° 0.596459'   W116° 57.345421'

The starting point is a California Division of Forestry fire station at the eastern base of Woodson Mountain, on SR 67, 3 miles north of Poway Road and 6 miles southwest of the SR 67 and SR 78 intersection in Ramona. Park on the wide east-side shoulder or on the narrower west-side shoulder of SR 67. Do not park on fire station property.

16 Iron Mountain

Trailhead Location: East of Poway in north-central San Diego County

Trail Use: Hiking, running, dog walking, mountain biking, horseback riding

Distance & Configuration: 6.4-mile out-and-back

Elevation Range: 1,611 feet at the start to 2,696 feet at the summit

Facilities: Restrooms and drinking water at the trailhead parking area

Highlights: A leisurely, seldom-steep ascent; ocean-to-mountain vistas as you approach the summit

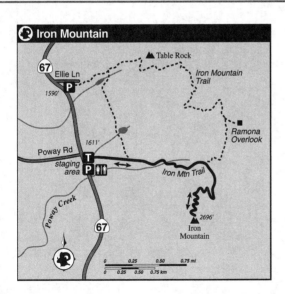

DESCRIPTION

Poway's Iron Mountain thrusts its conical, chaparral-clad summit nearly 2,700 feet above sea level, a height that is frequently well above the low-lying coastal haze. On many a crystalline winter day, the summit offers a sweeping, 360-degree panorama from glistening ocean to blue mountains and back to the ocean again. The main trail to the summit, 3.2 miles one way, is smoothly graded and hardly falters in its steady elevation gain. All kinds of self-propelled travelers use this popular trail, though mountain bikers and equestrians aren't seen much. On pleasant weekends, hundreds of hikers converge on this trail for their morning exercise.

THE ROUTE

From the trailhead parking lot, head east on the wide and almost level Iron Mountain Trail, flanked initially on both sides by rows of planted trees. Ignore the trail branching left (north) and continue on the main trail to a spot about 1 mile into the hike, where the trail narrows and briefly dips to cross the bottom of a ravine. On the far side of the ravine you climb in earnest for a while, negotiating the steepest grade you'll encounter along the whole route.

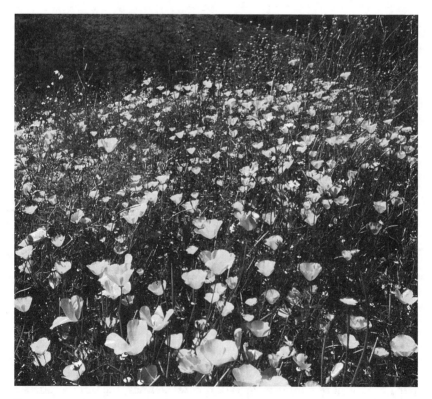

Poppies

At 1.5 miles you reach a saddle where you can turn left or right. Stay right (south) and commence a generally leisurely ascent through the low-growing sage scrub and chaparral shrubbery. Prior to the mid-1990s, the chaparral grew thick and tall here, sometimes high enough to form a tunnel overhead. Now, after two major wildfires, Iron Mountain's vegetation struggles to reach a climax phase, which takes at least 25–30 years of slow and steady growth.

After a definitive turn to the west, the ascent on the trail becomes steeper again, and final switchbacks take you back and forth across the ever-narrowing summit cone of Iron Mountain. On the boulders at the top, you will see a massive, pier-mounted telescope (no coins required) thoughtfully placed so anyone can scan the near and far horizons. You also may see a visitor register—a notebook stuffed with hundreds of written comments. When you are ready to return, go back the same way you came. (You can note a northern loop for your return on the accompanying map, but it adds 3 miles and several severe up-and-down pitches, so it is beyond the parameters of this guidebook.)

TO THE TRAILHEAD
GPS Coordinates: N32° 58.694222'   W116° 58.352938'
On I-15, about 15 miles north of central San Diego, exit at Scripps Poway Parkway. Follow Scripps Poway Parkway 9 miles east to its end at State Route 67. Turn left on SR 67 and drive 2 miles north to the traffic light at Poway Road. The 100-space Iron Mountain staging area and trailhead lies on the right. On weekends, this parking lot may fill up; overflow parking is allowed along the SR 67 shoulder.

17 Lake Poway Loop

Trailhead Location: Eastern Poway

Trail Use: Hiking, dog walking, running, mountain biking, horseback riding

Distance & Configuration: 2.4-mile loop trail

Elevation Range: 760–1,100 feet

Facilities: Water, restrooms, and picnic areas at the start

Highlights: Heart-pumping exercise while circumnavigating a scenic reservoir

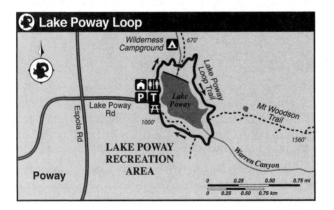

DESCRIPTION

Like most of San Diego County's water reservoirs, Lake Poway stores water imported through aqueducts from the Colorado River and from Northern California. Luckily, the city of Poway included a strong recreational element in the plan for the reservoir, which resulted in a wealth of recreational opportunities for the lake and its surroundings: picnicking, hiking, boating, fishing, and group camping.

The looping trail around Lake Poway serves two purposes: It's an excellent exercise trail for runners and walkers, with a good mixture of flats, gentle hills, and a few fairly steep switchbacks. It is also an interpretive trail, with a leaflet (available at the lake entrance or park office)

keyed to numbered posts along way. On the trail, you'll pass through four distinct plant communities: sage scrub, chaparral, oak woodland, and riparian woodland.

THE ROUTE

Find the Lake Poway Loop Trail just beyond the lake entrance, to the left of the park office and concession building. The trail follows the west shoreline to as far as the rock-fill dam, descends to a creek crossing, and soon reaches a dirt maintenance road. Turn left (north) and stay with that road for about 100 yards, where you will see the Lake Poway Loop Trail continuing on the right. (At that juncture, if you want, you can make a short side trip down to the Wilderness Campground, a walk-in or ride-in site for backpackers and equestrians. Tables at vacant sites can be used for picnicking.)

Follow the loop trail as it resumes climbing generally east, away from the dirt road. By way of a lengthy zigzag and a couple of smaller wiggles in the trail, you gain a slope above the east buttress of the Lake Poway Dam. Press on, traversing easily around the east shoreline, and note the junction of the Mount Woodson Trail on the left. Keep going straight, circling around the south arm of the lake, and arrive at the lawn area just shy of where you started the loop hike.

TO THE TRAILHEAD
GPS Coordinates: N33° 0.408540'   W117° 0.807481'
About 25 miles north of central San Diego, exit I-15 at Rancho Bernardo Road in Rancho Bernardo; go east. Rancho Bernardo Road becomes Espola Road as you enter Poway's city limits. Espola starts to curve south after about 3 miles. Drive a total of 4 miles from I-15 to reach Lake Poway Road. Turn left (east) there, and drive 0.5 mile to the Lake Poway Recreation Area, where plenty of parking space is available.

18 Blue Sky Ecological Reserve

Trailhead Location: Northern Poway

Trail Use: Hiking, dog walking, running, horseback riding

Distance & Configuration: 5-mile out-and-back

Elevation Range: 703 feet at the start to 1,350 feet at Ramona Reservoir

Facilities: Portable toilet at the trailhead and 1 mile in

Highlights: Dense riparian and oak woodlands, as well as scenic views from Ramona Reservoir Dam

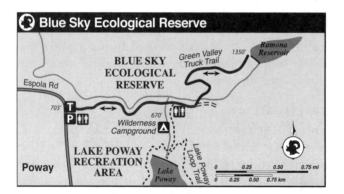

DESCRIPTION

The 700-acre Blue Sky Ecological Reserve near Poway protects one of the finest examples of riparian (streamside) vegetation in Southern California. As one of the most popular of the 119 California Department of Fish and Game wildlife reserves in the state, much attention here is focused on nature education as well as habitat preservation. Motorized vehicles and mountain bikes are banned, so you'll be assured of peace and quiet, and more frequent wildlife sightings, as you stroll along.

After a wet winter, usually by March, the reserve landscape turns an almost unbelievably bright shade of green. Mosses, ferns, annual grasses, and fresh new shrub growth coats everything, even the rocks. Wildflowers appear in great numbers by about April and start to fade by June, after the grasses have bleached to a straw-yellow color. More than 100 kinds of wildflowers have been identified here in a single year.

THE ROUTE

From the trailhead, follow the unpaved Green Valley Truck Trail along the south bank of a creek. Traffic noise disappears, and frogs entertain you with their guttural serenades. Live oaks spread their limbs overhead, casting pools of shade, while willows, sycamores, and lush thickets of poison oak cluster along the creek itself.

On the left, about 0.3 mile out, a side trail, parallel to the main trail, diverges toward the creek itself. There you can spot tadpoles, frogs, and perhaps other amphibious creatures. A narrower path takes you back to the truck trail. The sheer volume of poison-oak growth off of the main truck-trail route cannot be overemphasized; learn to recognize the plant's leaves-of-three pattern, and keep your pets well away!

Note: At 1 mile, a trail branching right (south) heads uphill to join the trail system of the Lake Poway Recreation Area (see hike 17, page 62). About 0.2 mile farther on the main road, where you will see power lines overhead, there's a major split. The left branch (Green Valley Truck Trail) fords the creek and starts climbing, as do you, a dry south-facing slope toward the Ramona Reservoir Dam. In the next 1.3 miles of steady ascent, you gain about 700 feet of elevation and enjoy an ever-expanding view of inland San Diego County's mix of suburban development and open space. If it's a hot summer day, you might want to forego for the time being that last 1.3 miles, which offers little or no shade.

Once you reach the dam and reservoir, you can turn around and return on the same route—downhill all the way.

TO THE TRAILHEAD

GPS Coordinates: N33° 0.948243'   W117° 1.411743'

Exit I-15 at Rancho Bernardo Road and go east. Rancho Bernardo Road becomes Espola Road as you enter the Poway city limits. Espola curves south after about 3 miles. The Blue Sky Ecological Reserve entrance is on the left, just after the curve, 3.4 miles from I-15.

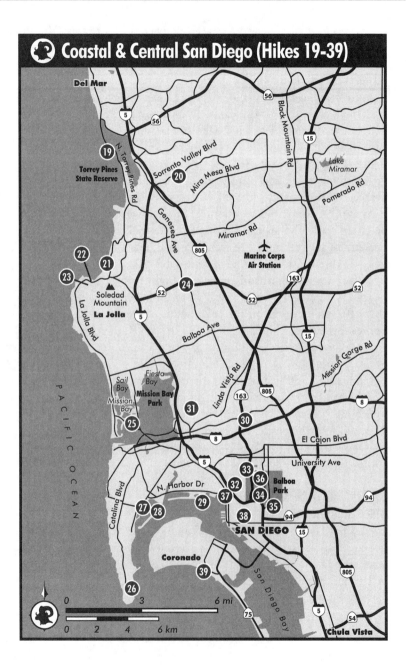

Coastal & Central San Diego (Hikes 19-39)

Del Mar

Torrey Pines
State Reserve

Sorrento Valley Blvd

Mira Mesa Blvd

Black Mountain Rd

Lake
Miramar

Pomerado Rd

N. Torrey Pines Rd

Genesee Ave

Miramar Rd

Marine Corps
Air Station

Soledad
Mountain

La Jolla

La Jolla Blvd

Balboa Ave

Mission Gorge Rd

Sail
Bay

Fiesta
Bay

Mission Bay
Park

Mission
Bay

Linda Vista Rd

El Cajon Blvd

University Ave

N. Harbor Dr

Balboa
Park

Catalina Blvd

SAN DIEGO

PACIFIC OCEAN

Coronado

San Diego Bay

Chula Vista

0   3   6 mi
0   2   4   6 km

COASTAL & CENTRAL SAN DIEGO

Regional Overview

Urban San Diego's landscape differs from that of most other densely populated major cities. Outside the compact downtown district, the city is a vast collection of distinct neighborhoods, some hugging the coast and others spreading inland.

San Diego's predominant canyon, mesa, and river valley topography ensures that not every acre of the city could, or would, be built upon. This of course is great news for urban hikers.

In addition to dozens of canyon-side open spaces, the city of San Diego has a long tradition of setting aside large tracts of land for use as city parks. One outstanding example is 1,200-acre Balboa Park, established in 1868 but not developed extensively unit the early 1900s. Another much more recent example is Mission Bay Park, with its 27 miles of shoreline. The latter's creation involved the conversion of mudflats into a modern-day, water-oriented recreational space.

Aside from these hiking and walking venues, opportunities abound for walks that highlight architectural and historic features. For example, relatively few locals, let alone tourists, are aware of the charming and intriguing footbridges spanning urban canyons just north of downtown. Even the core of downtown San Diego can offer up worthwhile viewing that simply would be missed if experienced by any conveyance other than on foot.

Central San Diego's proximity to the ocean goes hand-in-hand with year-round mild weather conditions. Another plus for hiking—on nearly all of the routes within this section—is that access to drinking water is of little concern, thanks to the nearby availability of public facilities, along with restaurants and small cafés.

You may, no doubt, face parking challenges on several of the hikes included in this section. However, as appropriate, the profiles will give you tips on where to begin the walk near reasonable parking areas.

19 Torrey Pines State Reserve

Trailhead Location: Just south of Del Mar

Trail Use: Hiking, running

Distance & Configuration: 1–4 miles on looping and out-and-back trails

Elevation Range: Sea level to 350 feet

Facilities: Water and restrooms at the trailheads

Highlights: Magnificent ocean vistas, rare flora, and nearly perfect year-round climate

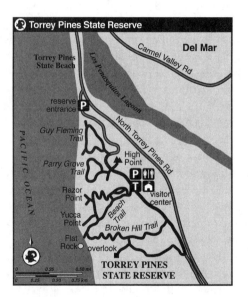

DESCRIPTION

The rare and beautiful Torrey pine trees atop the coastal bluffs south of Del Mar are as much a symbol of the Golden State as are the famed Monterey cypress trees native to California's central coast. Torrey pines grow naturally in only two places on earth: in and around Torrey Pines State Reserve and on Santa Rosa Island, off Santa Barbara. Of the estimated 6,000 or fewer native Torrey pines, more than half grow within the boundaries of the main reserve and its detached extension area.

Torrey Pines State Reserve would be botanically noteworthy even without its pines. More than 330 species of plants have been identified there so far. Sage scrub, chaparral, and salt marsh plant communities are present in various parts of the reserve.

If you're interested in identifying plants and wildflowers typical of the coast and coastal strip, the reserve is simply the best single place to go in San Diego County. Excellent interpretive facilities at the reserve's visitor center make this an easy task. Besides the exhibits, you can browse through several notebooks full of captioned photographs of common and rare plants within the reserve. You can also visit the native plant gardens surrounding the visitor building and at the head of the Parry Grove Trail.

If you visit the reserve a number of times during February–June, you'll be able to follow the succession of flowering as the spring season progresses. Wildflower maps, updated monthly, are often available.

THE ROUTE

Assuming you start at the reserve's main trailhead, a stone's throw from the visitor center, you'll have your choice of a variety of short- to moderate-length hikes, none involving more than 350 feet of elevation loss and gain.

For an overview of the entire area, you might first try the 100-yard-long trail to High Point, opposite the Parry Grove Trail, just north of the visitor center. You'll enjoy a panoramic view of the pine-clad uplands of the reserve, the ocean, and the flat, green Los Penasquitos Lagoon just east.

Next, you might head south on an antique concrete segment of the original Coast Highway, just south of the visitor center, and pick up the Broken Hill Trail. The two east branches of this trail wind through dense chaparral and connect with a spur trail leading to Broken Hill Overlook. You'll be able to step out (carefully) onto a precipitous fin of sandstone and peer over to see what looks like desert badlands. A third (west) branch of the Broken Hill Trail winds down a slope festooned with wildflowers and joins the Beach Trail at a point just above where the latter drops sharply to the beach.

The popular Beach Trail originates at the visitor center trailhead and heads downward toward the beach, intersecting with side trails to Yucca Point and Razor Point along the way. From these side destinations, you can peer nearly straight down to the sandy beach and surf. If you follow Beach Trail all the way down to the beach itself, any further travel would likely be blocked by high water during the highest tides, especially in winter, when strong wave action tends to strip sand away from the beach. At times of lower tides, and more often in summer and fall, you could head north along the sand and reach the reserve's entrance, 1 mile north.

Back to the Parry Grove and Guy Fleming loop trails, both north of the visitor center, you will wind among the most extensive groves of Torrey pines. Prolonged dry spells over the past 30 years or so—plus a resurgence of bark beetles—killed many of the large trees, especially those on the drier, south-facing slopes. Seedlings have been planted here and there in an effort to restore these groves to their former glory.

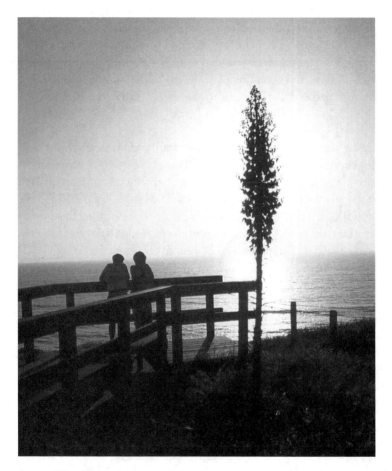

Sunset at Yucca Point

The Guy Fleming Trail is mostly flat, while the Parry Grove Trail starts with a steep descent on stair steps. In spring, the sunny slopes along the Guy Fleming Trail come alive with phantasmagoric wildflower displays. Fluttering in the sea breeze, the flowers put on quite a show as several vivid shades of color dynamically intermix with the more muted tones of earth, sea, and sky.

You can't picnic on any of the reserve's trails, but after you do your hiking, you can use the tables or the beach near the entrance. As with all hiking, do take water along on the trails. Also bring binoculars: The soaring ravens and the red-tailed and sparrow hawks are interesting to watch, as are humans lazily soaring about on paragliders. The gliders launch from the nearby Torrey Pines Glider Port.

TO THE TRAILHEAD

GPS Coordinates: N32° 55.196700'   W117° 15.177598'

Exit I-5 at Carmel Valley Road. Drive 1.5 miles west to the Coast Highway (signed Camino del Mar to the north and North Torrey Pines Road to the south). Go left and proceed 0.8 mile south to the Torrey Pines State Reserve parking lot on the right (fee charged), or find a parking spot for free along the Coast Highway. You also may enter the reserve entrance, pay the fee, and drive about 1 mile farther to the visitor center and main trailhead at the top of the coastal bluffs.

20 Los Penasquitos Canyon

Trailhead Location: East of Del Mar

Trail Use: Hiking, running, mountain biking, dog walking, horseback riding

Distance & Configuration: 5.5-mile out-and-back

Elevation Range: 35 feet at the start to 190 feet

Facilities: Restrooms at the trailhead

Highlights: A cascading waterfall following the winter rains

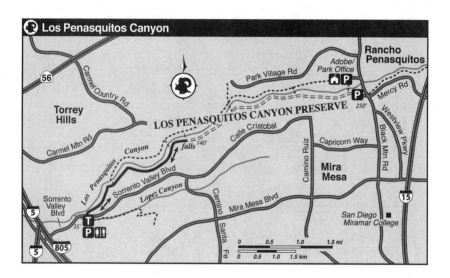

DESCRIPTION

Crickets sing and bullfrogs groan. A hawk alights upon a sycamore limb and then launches with outstretched wings to catch a puff of sea breeze moving up the canyon. A cottontail rabbit bounds across the trail and stops to take your measure with a sidelong stare. Los Penasquitos Creek, rejuvenated by winter rains, slips silently through a sparkling pool and darts noisily down multiple paths in the constriction known as "the falls."

Despite the miles of suburban development surrounding it, Los Penasquitos Canyon Preserve still retains its gentle, unself-conscious beauty. The preserve's 3,000 acres of San Diego city- and county-owned open space stretch for almost 7 miles between the I-5/I-805 merge and I-15, encompassing much of Los Penasquitos Creek and one of its tributaries, Lopez Canyon. Aside from historic dwellings and ruins dating back to the mid-1800s, the preserve hosts a trail system popular with every sort of self-propelled traveler.

The falls lie nearly at the midpoint of a 6-mile-long, unspoiled segment of Los Penasquitos Canyon; they are equally accessible from the east or the west via a wide pathway—the unpaved access road that ran the length of the canyon in its cattle-ranch days.

Here, we profile the west approach to the falls, which offers spacious views of the canyon bottom and hillsides, plus some of the finest springtime wildflower scenery to be found anywhere in San Diego County. If you're feeling adventurous, try this hike on a warm afternoon and evening: Plan to reach the falls by sunset, and return by the light of a full moon.

THE ROUTE

From your starting point at the preserve's west-side staging area and trailhead, follow the main trail going west underneath Sorrento Valley Boulevard and up broad and shallow Los Penasquitos Canyon. Sometimes fine springtime displays of lupine and owl's clover cover the steep, grassy slopes on the right. Wild radish, a plant introduced from Europe, often paints the lower slopes with shades of blue, white, and purple.

At about 0.7 mile, the trail comes close to the creek, and there's a creek crossing on the left leading to a singletrack trail on the far side. This is only the first of several minor side trails in the next several miles that link to pathways on the far bank. Your way, however, sticks to the main trail, which remains on the right (south) bank.

The main trail eventually climbs a small hill and then descends to more grassland, dotted with small trees and shrubs such as elderberry, live oak, laurel sumac, toyon, and gooseberry. Large sycamores and cottonwoods flank the creek to your left.

At about 2.5 miles into the hike, the trail starts curving up a chaparral-covered slope. Near the top, there's a wide spot with racks for securing bikes and a foot trail descending north to the falls area, where the Los Penasquitos stream has carved a narrow constriction into the bedrock.

When the flow of water is sufficient, typically January–May, water exuberantly cascades through here. Polished rock 10 feet up on either side testifies to its maximum depth in flood stage. The greenish-gray outcrops responsible for the cascading path of the water are a type of erosion-resistant metavolcanic rock (volcanic rock hardened by heat and pressure). When the weather is warm, be vigilant in the area around the falls since rattlesnakes may be out and about.

When it's time to return, use the same route you traveled to get here.

TO THE TRAILHEAD

GPS Coordinates: N32° 54.391923'   W117° 12.362337'

Exit I-805 at Mira Mesa Boulevard/Sorrento Valley Road. Take either I-805 frontage road (Sorrento Valley Road on the west side; Vista Sorrento Parkway on the east side) 1 mile north to Sorrento Valley Boulevard. Turn right and continue 1 mile east to a marked trailhead and staging area for Los Penasquitos Canyon Preserve, on the right.

21 La Jolla Shores

Trailhead Location: La Jolla

Trail Use: Hiking, running

Distance & Configuration: 2-mile out-and-back

Elevation Range: Sea level all the way

Facilities: Water and restrooms at Kellogg Park

Highlights: One of California's finest stretches of coastline, with sandy beach, dramatic sea bluffs, and tide pools, all within a short stretch

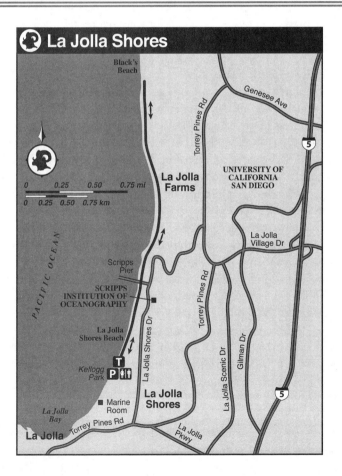

DESCRIPTION

For beachcombing, tidepool exploration, and all-over suntanning, La Jolla Shores Beach and the coastal stretch north of it can't be beat. It's important to note, though, that some of the better attributes of this environment aren't available at higher tides—typically 3 feet or more. In fact, the highest tides of up to 7 feet will limit your walk along the beach to only 0.5 mile each way, assuming you don't want to be swamped by waves. Extreme low tides (expressed on tide tables as 0 feet to -2 feet), on the other hand, are perfect for viewing marine life amid the rocky outcrops that lie at the lowest levels of the intertidal zone.

The timing of extreme low tides depends on the time of year. October–March, the extreme lows (which coincide with new and full moons) tend to occur during afternoon hours. April–September, similarly low tides are confined to the predawn hours—not great for those who value their sleep.

THE ROUTE

You'll begin walking on the beach adjacent to the grassy area known as Kellogg Park. Walk north on the sand, passing under the cliff-hugging buildings of Scripps Institution of Oceanography. The initial stretch of sand is gently shelving, extremely wide, and a pleasure to enjoy with bare feet during low-tide episodes. On the wet sand nearest the waves, you might catch shimmery reflections of Scripps Pier and looming Torrey Pines bluffs beyond.

You pass under Scripps Pier after about 0.5 mile. Just ahead, the cliffs on the right get taller and pinch in toward the water. You're on sandstone rocks and boulders now, wet and slippery near the waves and smooth and dry higher up, so put your shoes back on. The rocky tidepool area exposed during low tide is visibly wriggling with plant and animal life. The sea vegetation tends to move to and fro with the waves at the water's edge, while the sea creatures, including tiny fish, sea stars, shore and hermit crabs, and even octopuses, flit about at variable rates of speed. Please note that all species are protected here, and no collecting is allowed.

Near the end of the tidepools, notice the narrow finger, or *dike* in geologic parlance, of grayish volcanic rock stretching diagonally out to sea, toward the southwest. This is the only significant exposure of volcanic rock along San Diego County's coastline. It dates from some 11 million years ago, in the Miocene epoch, when a pulse of magma pushed its way up nearly to Earth's surface.

Right after you pass the dike, the sandy beach resumes, flanked by tall cliffs on the right and the crashing surf on the left. You might want to slip off your shoes again and enjoy the feel of the fine, clean sand underfoot. By that point, or not far ahead, you may notice that some beachgoers have doffed more than just shoes. You're now on Torrey Pines City Beach, also known as Black's Beach, San Diego's ever-popular nude bathing and sunbathing spot. The warmer the weather, the more skin is exposed here. So, for whatever reasons you want, you can either turn back here, for this 2-mile round-trip walk, or continue north for literally miles ahead. If you press on forward, do so *only* if you have checked the tide tables for *that day*. It is imperative that you remain mindful of any incoming higher tide that might swamp your return route.

TO THE TRAILHEAD
GPS Coordinates: N32° 51.472979'   W117° 15.405600'
From northbound I-5 or westbound State Route 52, take La Jolla Parkway west toward La Jolla. La Jolla Parkway merges into Torrey Pines Road. Immediately after, turn right onto La Jolla Shores Drive. Go five or six blocks north and turn left on narrow residential streets leading west to Kellogg Park, where a large parking lot lies in between two spacious grassy areas.

22 Coast Walk

Trailhead Location: La Jolla

Trail Use: Hiking, dog walking, running

Distance & Configuration: 1.5-mile out-and-back

Elevation Range: 100 feet at the start to sea level

Facilities: Water, restrooms, and commercial facilities in the village of La Jolla

Highlights: One of California's most famous and dramatic meldings of land and sea

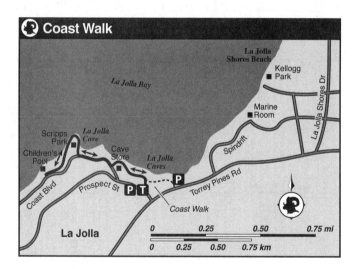

DESCRIPTION

You get a stunning perspective of La Jolla Bay and the sparkling La Jolla Shores coastline on this short walk along the cliff tops. You'll be walking directly above the La Jolla Caves, on or near the very brink of a 100-foot drop to the bay's calm surface. This fact should alert you to be watchful of small children, if you have any along.

THE ROUTE

From the Prospect Street cul-de-sac parking spaces, find the public-access stairs and path leading toward a trail paralleling the brink. The trail leads right a short distance to two obscure public parking spaces at the west end of a paved street signed COAST WALK (an alternative place to park your car) and leads left toward La Jolla Cove. Stay left and pass below the backyards of several palatial houses, all the while enjoying a spacious panorama of the blue ocean.

After only 0.2 mile, you arrive at a grove of graceful, planted Torrey pine trees. A fenced viewpoint lies below on the right, and the Cave Store lies immediately to the left. The Cave Store, which has gone by different names in the past and dates from 1902, features a 144-step staircase down a tunnel leading to the westernmost of the series of La Jolla Caves—Sunny Jim Cave.

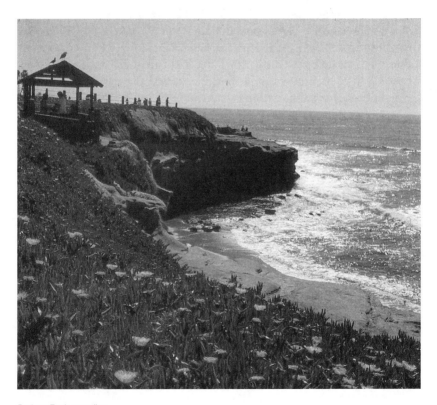

Scripps Park coastline

Press on, continuing downhill on a sidewalk now, to the pocket beach of La Jolla Cove and the adjoining grassy space known as Scripps Park. Along the way, you can watch swimmers, snorkelers, and divers below as they float or glide through the often-glassy water. Once in Scripps Park, simply follow the curving sidewalk that stays close to the pounding surf, just below. After 5 or 10 minutes on the sidewalk, you'll arrive at the ever-popular Children's Pool breakwater and pocket beach, which has gained much attention over the years on account of its wholesale colonization by harbor seals.

After gawking at the seals, which are separated from the tourist crowds by a rope barrier, you can either head back the way you came, or try a different tack: Head uphill, two blocks inland, to Prospect Street. Prospect Street is La Jolla's most elegant shopping-boutique thoroughfare, and it can take you straight back to your starting point.

TO THE TRAILHEAD
GPS Coordinates: N32° 50.879760'   W117° 16.078019'
From northbound I-5 or westbound State Route 52, take La Jolla Parkway west toward La Jolla. La Jolla Parkway merges into Torrey Pines Road after 1.3 miles. Continue west on Torrey Pines Road another 1 mile to Prospect Street. Turn right, and within a short block, find the short cul-de-sac on the right with free public parking spaces.

23 Soledad Mountain

Trailhead Location: La Jolla

Trail Use: Hiking, dog walking, running, bicycling

Distance & Configuration: 6-mile out-and-back

Elevation Range: 100 feet at the start to 811 feet at the top of Soledad Park

Facilities: No restrooms along the route; drinking water at Soledad Park

Highlights: World-class coast-to-mountain vistas and residential mansions to admire

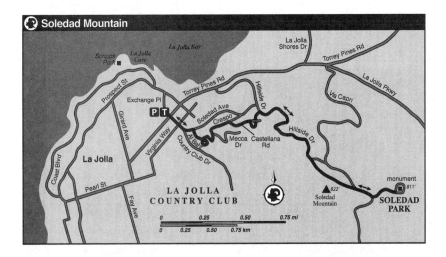

DESCRIPTION

Follow this eclectic route for a unique look at La Jolla, from the edge of the village's commercial center to 811 feet of elevation atop Soledad Mountain. Cyclists using road or mountain bikes can follow this same route, but beware: There are some tough uphill stretches here, suitable only for bikes with very low gears or a willingness to walk the bike in some spots.

THE ROUTE

Set off by going south (uphill) on Exchange Place. Busy Torrey Pines Road lies right ahead, and you may need to use the traffic light at Prospect, one block away, to cross safely on foot. Continue up Exchange Place and into one of La Jolla's serene older neighborhoods.

Within three short blocks, Exchange Place splits into Country Club Drive on the right and Soledad Avenue on the left. Take the latter. After one block on Soledad, go right on Al Bahr Drive. On Al Bahr, follow a curious curlicue under and then over a gracefully arched bridge. At the top of the curlicue, turn right on Crespo Street.

After completing a hairpin turn on Crespo, look for the intersection of Mecca Drive on the right. An optional but worthwhile side trip (that adds only 0.3 mile round-trip) to this 6-mile walk takes you higher up this dead-end narrow lane to a startling drop-off that offers airy and unobstructed views of La Jolla Bay and the North County coastline. Here you can enjoy the same stupendous views afforded from some of La Jolla's finest homes.

Back down (or ahead, if you did not venture up Mecca Drive) on Crespo Street, look for the inconspicuous intersection of Castellana Road,

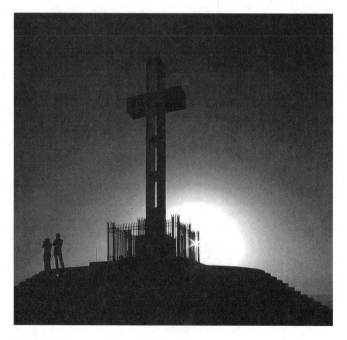

Soledad Park cross

where you veer right. Just ahead, you can visit a hidden overlook at the point where Puente Road, a stubby cul-de-sac, passes over Castellana Road on an arched bridge similar to the one seen earlier. From there, tall trees frame a view of tile rooftops and La Jolla Bay.

Next, back up a little and follow Castellana as it goes under the bridge and descends to meet Hillside Drive. Turn right on Hillside and follow its steep and winding course upward along the north slope of Soledad Mountain. Make no turns; just stay on the main winding drive, which is flanked by cliff-hanging mansions, some of them perched on postage-stamp-size, outrageously expensive view lots. In between these choice properties are jaw-dropping vistas of the coastline curving to the north.

On ahead you'll come to a sturdy, unlocked pipe gate. Go through it, maintaining your course upward on the old (now closed to traffic) road-bed of Hillside Drive. After some huffing and puffing and ever-widening views of the inland landscape, you reach Via Capri. From there you have only another 5 minutes or so of not-so-pleasant road-shoulder walking to reach Soledad Park.

A tall Easter cross still stands at the high point of Soledad Park, despite decades of controversy centered on the legality of its continued existence. A veteran's memorial installation now surrounds the cross to serve as a memorial to fallen soldiers and sailors.

The view from the base of the Easter cross is panoramic, except to the west where a slightly higher ridge—the true summit of Soledad Mountain—rises. In every other direction, you can check out the seemingly infinite spread of urbia/suburbia spreading east toward the distant mountain crest and the arterial pattern of wide freeways and major streets curving this way and that. In the south, skyscrapers in downtown San Diego loom, Mission Bay sparkles in the sunshine, and Point Loma juts like a southward pointing finger into the blue Pacific.

After enjoying the summit view, head back downhill, returning the same way you came.

TO THE TRAILHEAD

GPS Coordinates: N32° 50.769417' W117° 16.200721'
From northbound I-5 or westbound State Route 52, take La Jolla Parkway west toward La Jolla. La Jolla Parkway merges into Torrey Pines Road after 1.3 miles. Continue west on Torrey Pines Road another 1 mile to Prospect Street and turn right. Within a short block, turn left on Park Row. Park at or near the intersection of Park Row and Exchange Place, just ahead.

24 Marian Bear Memorial Park

Trailhead Location: Inland from La Jolla

Trail Use: Hiking, dog walking, running, mountain biking

Distance & Configuration: Up to 6 miles (double out-and-backs)

Elevation Range: 60–220 feet

Facilities: Water, restrooms, and picnic tables at the start; restrooms and picnic tables near Regents Road parking

Highlights: Canopies of live oak and sycamore trees, plus a trickling stream

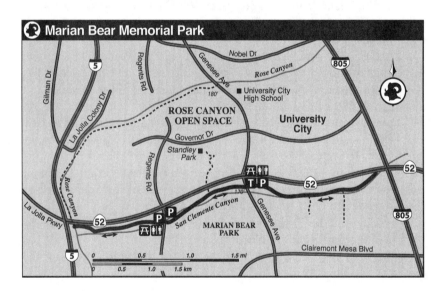

DESCRIPTION

Eastbound in the right lane of State Route 52, the San Clemente Canyon Freeway, you can look down upon a long, slender, almost unbroken swath of natural vegetation: massive sycamores, stately live oaks, climbing vines, and tangled shrubs. This is one of San Diego County's best examples of riparian (stream-loving) vegetation, and it's very rare in Southern California. Only 0.2% of San Diego County's land area consists of riparian vegetation.

Much of San Clemente Canyon and several of its steep finger (small tributary) canyons are included within the boundaries of Marian Bear Memorial Park, an area set aside by the city of San Diego as natural open space. Facilities include parking areas, picnic tables, and restrooms off Regents Road and Genesee Avenue and resting benches elsewhere. You won't get completely away from freeway traffic noise while hiking here, but you can minimize the disturbance by arriving early on Saturdays, Sundays, and holidays.

An old roadbed—today a trail of variable width—follows the canopy of trees along the canyon's seasonal stream. The path stretches about 3 miles, is almost flat, and crosses the streambed four times. In summer these crossings simply mean a hop and a skip across cobblestones, but in winter some shallow-water wading may be necessary.

The east end of the park (between Genesee Avenue and I-805) offers the prettiest vegetation, the densest shade, and a proliferation of poison-oak vines that are adjacent to but not encroaching upon the trail. Beginning about October, the leaves of the poison oak turn bright red in pleasing complement to the evergreen live oaks and the yellows and oranges of the sycamores and willows.

THE ROUTE

Starting from the Genesee Avenue Trailhead, you can travel as far as about 1 mile east toward I-805 or about 2 miles west toward I-5, all the while staying parallel to the freeway. That makes a round-trip of 6 miles if you go both directions. In addition, a number of small side trails dart upward to hook up with neighborhoods to the north and south. On the west side of Marian Bear Memorial Park, a trail connects San Clemente Canyon to the next major open-space canyon area to the north, the Rose Canyon Open Space.

TO THE TRAILHEAD

GPS Coordinates: N32° 50.749083'   W117° 12.045600'

Exit SR 52 at Genesee Avenue, which is 2 miles east of I-5 and 1 mile west of I-805. Go south on Genesee. The principal trailhead for Marian Bear Memorial Park is on the east side of Genesee, just south of the freeway.

25 Circling Sail Bay

Trailhead Location: Mission Beach

Trail Use: Hiking, running, dog walking, bicycling, in-line skating

Distance & Configuration: 5-mile loop

Elevation Range: Sea level up to 50 feet on major bridges

Facilities: A major commercial street, Mission Boulevard, lies one block west in the early part of the hike, so water and restrooms are handy at frequent intervals in the first half of the walk.

Highlights: A circumnavigation of picture-perfect, sail-flecked Sail Bay, the most scenic arm of Mission Bay

DESCRIPTION

More than a decade's worth of public improvements have literally paved the way for pedestrians, cyclists, Segway riders, and skaters traveling along the curving shoreline of west Mission Bay and its upper extremity, Sail Bay. Concrete paths smooth enough for roller skating go right along the bay shoreline, barely high enough to avoid being swamped at the highest tides. To complete a loop around Sail Bay you have to pass over open water three times on sidewalks that accompany busy roads, but at least those sidewalks are generously wide and offer some fine views of the blue waters of Mission Bay and the colorful neighborhoods that surround it.

THE ROUTE

From your starting point at Dana Landing, follow the sidewalk going west toward West Mission Bay Drive. Some wooden stairs will take you directly to the sidewalk that accompanies the roadway. Head west across the bridge over Mission Bay's main channel, and after another 0.5 mile veer right on Bayside Walk, a concrete pathway striking north along the shore of Mission Bay.

Bayside Walk differs enormously from the paralleling Ocean Front Walk, which borders the sand at Mission Beach only three blocks west. The popular Ocean Front Walk is often filled with cyclists, skaters, and pedestrians dodging each other, showing off, and gawking. If that's what you'd like to experience, then head over that way. Otherwise stay on the much more sedate Bayside Walk, which squeezes between wall-to-wall beach cottages on the left and the sandy shore of the bay on the right. You pass Santa Clara Point on the right, a popular launching spot for small sailing craft.

After more than a mile on Bayside Walk, you start curving east on newer and smoother slabs of concrete set low in the sand. Right after the Catamaran Resort Hotel, you gently climb and descend for nearly 100

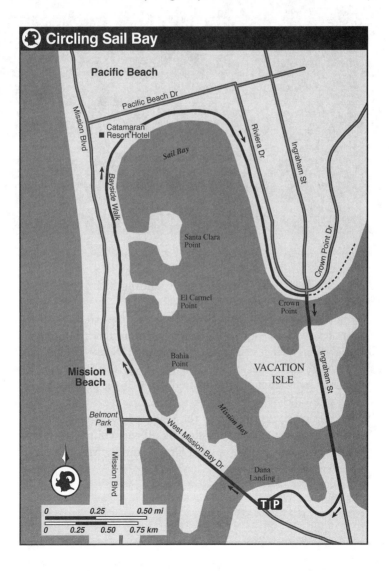

Circling Sail Bay

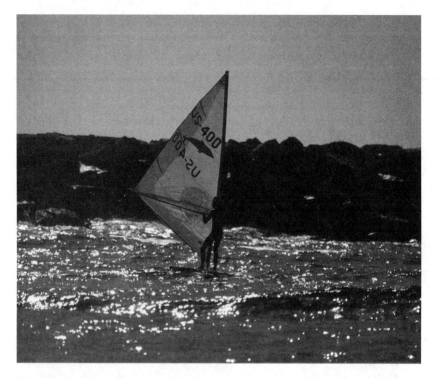

Sailboarding on Mission Bay

yards over the Briarfield Cove Bridge, spanning a tiny tidal slough at Sail Bay's north end.

Continue curving past a grassy mini-park on the left and farther into Riviera Shores, which features multistory condominium buildings overlooking the water. When you reach the Ingraham Street Bridge, don't go straight under it but rather climb the stairway to the left, up to Riviera Drive at street level. Swing right on Ingraham Street and head south on Ingraham's sidewalk.

In the next mile, you pass over the two long, separate bridges spanning Mission Bay, staying on the sidewalk all the while. On the far side of the second bridge, veer right toward Dana Landing Marina, and return to your parked car.

TO THE TRAILHEAD

GPS Coordinates: N32° 46.025820'   W117° 14.342637'

Exit I-8 at West Mission Bay Drive. Head north on a bridge over the San Diego River. As you approach the landscaped interchange ahead, go around the cloverleaf ramp to the right, following signs for the continuation of West Mission Bay Drive. Turn right at the first traffic light and park your car in any lot at or near the Dana Landing Marina.

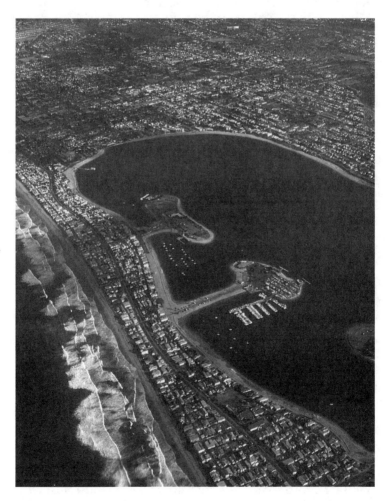

Sail Bay

26 Bayside Trail

Trailhead Location: Tip of Point Loma

Trail Use: Hiking, running

Distance & Configuration: 2-mile out-and-back

Elevation Range: 420 feet at trailhead to 90 feet at bottom of trail

Facilities: Water and restrooms at the adjacent Cabrillo National Monument Visitor Center

Highlights: The most comprehensive Pacific Ocean and San Diego Bay views you can get—short of flying

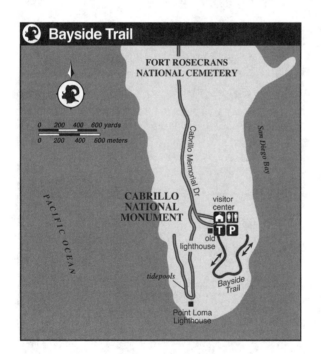

DESCRIPTION

The long, south-pointing peninsula of Point Loma and the spectacular curving shoreline of San Diego Bay are two of the principal elements responsible for San Diego's legendary beauty. Most of the south half of the Point Loma peninsula is reserved for military uses. Perched on its end, centered on the highest promontory, is one of America's smallest (144 acres) national monuments, Cabrillo National Monument. Because of its location adjacent to the tourist-happy city of San Diego, Cabrillo is consistently ranked as one of the two busiest national monuments in the country.

Hikers can enjoy the view-rich Bayside Trail that begins at the historic Old Point Loma Lighthouse atop Point Loma and offers an incomparable view of the city of San Diego and its watery environs. Amid the sweet-pungent sage scrub and chaparral vegetation, you get an eyeful of San Diego Bay, the Silver Strand, and the gleaming downtown skyline. You'll double your pleasure if you walk this trail on a crystal-clear day, fairly typical of the late-fall and winter seasons in San Diego.

THE ROUTE

From the Cabrillo National Monument parking lot, first head south (uphill) to the lighthouse. Just east of the lighthouse, pick up the signed Bayside Trail, which begins with 0.3 mile of descending pavement. Make a hard left turn and travel the remaining 0.7 mile of gravel-surfaced trail. You descend east, losing most of the remaining elevation, and then turn north. Large metal interpretive plaques have been installed along this latter part of the trail, detailing the cultural and natural history of the area.

Point Loma's bay slope is honeycombed with the ruins of a World War II defense system of mortars, observation bunkers, generators, and searchlights. You will see some of these remains along the trail. At the point where the trail ends (or rather runs into off-limits U.S. Navy property), you'll still be about 90 feet in elevation above San Diego Bay's surface. This is a good place to observe the sailboats and ships maneuvering in and out of the bay's narrow entrance. There are also aerial acrobatics to watch, courtesy of gulls, terns, and pelicans—plus, possibly, aircraft taking off and landing at the North Island Naval Air Station across the bay.

Return to the lighthouse the same way you came, uphill all the way. Tempting as it may be, don't take shortcuts: The vegetation is easily trampled and the soil eroded by one footprint too many. Besides, off-trail exploration is strictly forbidden within the national monument.

Back at the Old Point Loma Lighthouse, consider taking a look inside, where you are allowed to climb partway up the spiral staircase. Not much has changed appearance-wise from the structure's days as a working lighthouse, 1855–1891. Just south of the lighthouse a whale-watching overlook offers a spectacular view west over what seems like the whole Pacific

Ocean. December–February, migrating gray whales are commonly spotted swimming close to the shore. Binoculars help a lot in this endeavor.

TO THE TRAILHEAD

GPS Coordinates: N32° 40.437899'   W117° 14.406302'
From I-5 or I-8, at the interchange where the two freeways meet, take the Rosecrans Boulevard exit. Proceed 3 miles southwest on Rosecrans to Canon Street on the right. Drive uphill on Canon Street, which merges with Catalina Boulevard after 1.2 miles. Keep going south on Catalina, past a military gate (open to the public from 9 a.m. to roughly sunset), and finally into Cabrillo National Monument at the road's end. Pay the fee at the entrance checkpoint, and head for the large parking lot beyond.

27 La Playa & Point Loma

Trailhead Location: Point Loma

Trail Use: Hiking, running, limited dog walking

Distance & Configuration: 2.5-mile loop

Elevation Range: Sea level to 170 feet

Facilities: The Point Loma business district is nearby.

Highlights: Fine homes and San Diego Bay and marina views

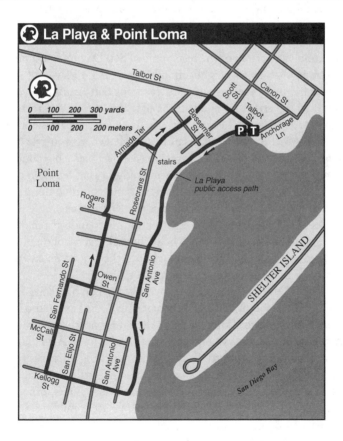

DESCRIPTION

This circular route follows a publicly accessible bayside pathway and rambles along narrow residential lanes in a San Diego Bay–facing neighborhood of Point Loma. Along the way, you'll pass two of the city's most celebrated marinas, the San Diego and Southwestern yacht clubs. Near the end, at an obscure opening between two hillside houses, you enjoy a view with a sense of déjà vu: the secret spot where local postcard photographers produce some of their most famous images. You can enjoy the bay-shore part of this ramble with your leashed dog too—but not 9 a.m.–5 p.m., when the path is closed to pets.

THE ROUTE

From Anchorage Lane, head down the sandy, bayside path. Shelter Island, to the left, fringed with yachts, extends nearly parallel with your path. The island is a peninsula, really—an artificial barrier island made of sand and mud dredged from the bottom of the bay. Some of San Diego's finest homes lie to your right, in the pocket neighborhood known as La Playa.

After about 0.5 mile, the bayside pathway joins San Antonio Avenue. Follow this residential street for about three blocks and then return to the shore, a sandy intertidal beach flecked with shells, when the pavement runs out. Continue on to the end of that sandy stretch, where you reach the boundary fence of the U.S. Naval Reservation that occupies a big chunk of the Point Loma peninsula ahead. Simply turn right at that fence, and follow Kellogg Street west. Cross Rosecrans Street and continue uphill into one of Point Loma's most attractive and quiet residential areas.

Two blocks past Rosecrans, turn right on San Fernando Street. Pepper trees lining both sides of the street help conceal several opulent residences. Tall pines and eucalyptus trees reach into the sky, often snagging the cottony morning fog creeping over Point Loma's ridgeline.

A right turn on Owen Street followed by a left turn on San Elijo Street takes you to a T-intersection at Rogers Street. Turn left (west) and walk about 30 feet to find a narrow, dirt pathway threading north between two homes. After a short passage, you'll reach the dead end of Armada Terrace. Follow Armada north toward Talbot Street, catching glimpses of the city, the bay, and the yacht basin. Many classic, long-lens photographs of San Diego's downtown skyline have been captured hereabouts, especially between two residential properties that happen to have a public stairway descending between them. From the top of that stairway, the panoramic view includes hundreds of boats at anchor, directly in front of a wide patch of San Diego Bay, plus the toothy downtown San Diego skyline.

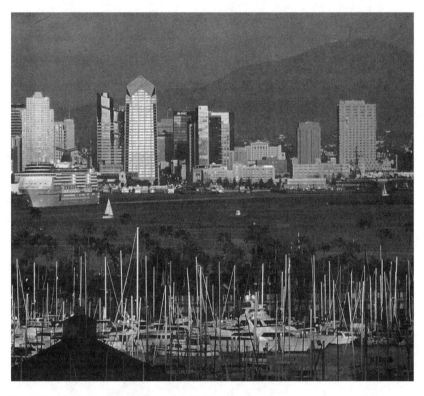

View of downtown San Diego Bay from Armada Terrace

Take that same public stairway down to Rosecrans, and turn left when you reach it. (If you overlook or pass the stairs, use the next street, Bessemer Street, to reach Rosecrans.) Head north to Talbot Street, turn right, and within two blocks you'll be back at your parked car.

TO THE TRAILHEAD
GPS Coordinates: N32° 43.147681'   W117° 13.872542'
From I-5 or I-8, at the interchange where the two freeways meet, take the Rosecrans Boulevard exit. Proceed 3 miles southwest on Rosecrans to Canon Street. Turn left, drive three blocks, and turn right on Anchorage Lane. Go one block and park on the street, where Anchorage Lane becomes Talbot Street. A sign marks the start of a bayside pathway here.

28 Shelter Island

Trailhead Location: Point Loma

Trail Use: Running, night hiking

Distance & Configuration: 2-mile out-and-back

Elevation Range: Sea level throughout

Facilities: Drinking water, public restrooms, hotels, and restaurants throughout

Highlights: Witness San Diego's best sunrises, sunsets, and moonrises from Shelter Island's shoreline pathway.

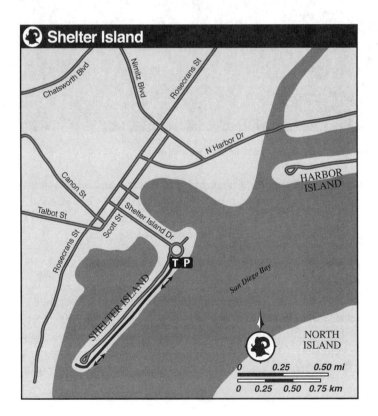

DESCRIPTION

If, as a San Diegan, Shelter Island seems overly familiar to you, then try visiting this artificial island (or shall we say peninsula, which is technically more correct) at either the opening or the closing of any clear day. That's when magic occurs with the sun, and sometimes the moon.

First, let's mention some of the island's history and its features. From its origins as a muddy shoal, the island was built up as dry land through dredging operations in San Diego Bay in the 1930s and '40s. By the 1950s, development was under way, and the island assumed its present persona as a shoreline resort destination, with hotels, restaurants, marinas, and a linear stretch of parkland about a mile long that features one of the finest walking paths in town. Over the years, several pieces of public art have been installed alongside that path. They include the *Tunaman's Memorial* (a bronze sculpture of tuna fishers in action), the *Yokohama Friendship Bell* (a gift from the city of Yokohama, Japan), and two monumental sculptures at opposite ends of the island—*Pacific Portal* and *Pearl of the Pacific*—by local artist James Hubbell.

Shelter Island's maritime eye candy includes hundreds of boats at anchor, most of which are associated with the Silvergate, Southwestern, and San Diego yacht clubs. The shoreline is a favored spot for viewing Fourth of July fireworks over San Diego Bay and December's holiday lights boat parade.

From an astronomical standpoint, Shelter Island is visually sweet because it lies 3–4 miles due west of, and straight across the bay from, downtown San Diego's skyscrapers. Try taking a walk on the island path during either sunrise or sunset. In March and April, and also in September and October, the rising sun's rays thread through gaps between the distant buildings. The setting sun during those same months sends reflections off of any glass or metal surface in the downtown area, and the skyline burns with a fiery glow.

Every time there's a full moon, the moon's act of rising in the east is coincident (or nearly coincident) with the sun's setting. Again, for the months of March, April, September, and October, the rising full moon at sunset is closely aligned over the skyline. Barring low clouds or fog, the scene is a spectacle to behold.

THE ROUTE

From Shelter Island's traffic circle, on the side of the island facing downtown San Diego, pick up the shoreline sidewalk curving southeast past a public fishing pier. In the next 1 mile, enjoy the superlative views and walk along with all sorts of locals and tourists. Grassy spaces and picnic

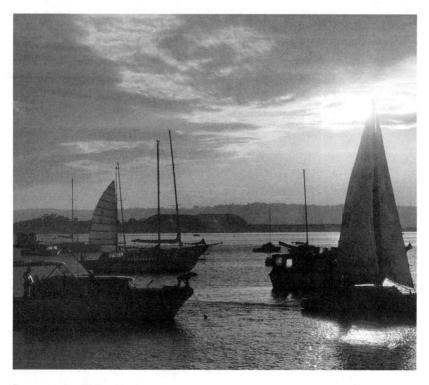

Boats at anchor, Shelter Island

tables, all very popular for family get-togethers on fair-weather week-ends, flank the sidewalk.

When you reach the far end of the island, turn around and return, enjoying the same great vistas from the reverse perspective.

TO THE TRAILHEAD

GPS Coordinates: N32° 43.005960'   W117° 13.352938'

From I-5 or I-8, at the interchange where the two freeways meet, take the Rosecrans Boulevard exit. Proceed 3 miles southwest on Rosecrans to Shelter Island Drive. Turn left and drive 0.7 mile to the traffic circle on Shelter Island. Parking spaces are abundant either on the street or in the large public parking lots just past the traffic circle.

29 Harbor Island

Trailhead Location: Next to San Diego International Airport

Trail Use: Hiking, running, dog walking, night hiking

Distance & Configuration: 3-mile out-and-back from the island end-to-end

Elevation Range: Sea level throughout

Facilities: Drinking water, public restrooms, hotels, and restaurants throughout

Highlights: Unbeatable bay and skyline views

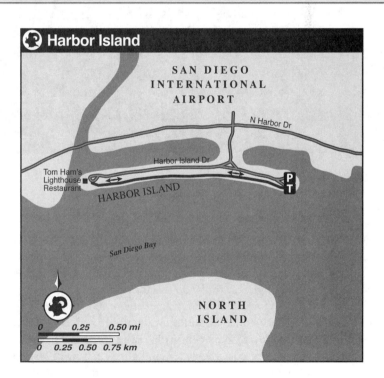

DESCRIPTION

Harbor Island, like Shelter Island (hike 28, page 96), is an artificial, T-shaped peninsula lined with hotels, restaurants, small-boat marinas, and a grassy

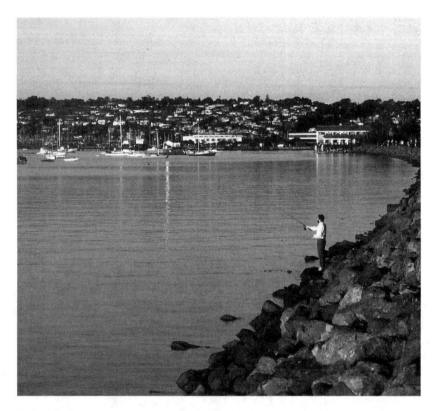

Harbor Island

linear park fronting the waters of San Diego Bay. On the concrete sidewalk running the length of linear park, you'll meet plenty of other people hanging out on benches, fishing from the sidewalk, watching for birds (which includes at least one resident great blue heron), and strolling or jogging along the path itself. Bikes and skates are not allowed on the path, though they are allowed to mix with the light car traffic on the adjacent roadway.

At most any time of year and almost any time of day, the views from Harbor Island are at least handsome and at most stunning. Westbound, the panorama includes the Point Loma peninsula rising above the bay waters, aircraft carriers at anchor across the water, and a steady flow of large and small vessels cruising in or out of the bay. The eastbound vantage includes downtown San Diego's skyline, shadowy in the morning mist, gleaming in the golden light of afternoon, and often reflecting in the water. Behind the skyline, the higher mountaintops of San Diego County are visible on clear days. Off to the right, the San Diego–Coronado Bridge executes a low arc over the horizon.

THE ROUTE

Starting from Harbor Island's east end, follow the bayside sidewalk west. The gently curving sidewalk, flanked by benches and a grassy strip of variable widths, ends 1.5 miles later, at Tom Ham's Lighthouse Restaurant on the island's west end. To return, simply retrace your steps. With the right timing, you could face the setting sun on the outbound leg, and the rising full moon on the return leg.

On evenings April–September, on nights when the moon is full, the rising moon appears right behind or nearly behind the skyline, particularly as seen from Tom Ham's. Savor the moment as the pumpkinlike moon silently launches itself right over the twilight-bathed city. (There is, however, one caveat about evenings on Harbor Island. Coastal San Diego commonly experiences "May gray" and "June gloom." These seasonal low-overcast conditions spoil any view of the setting sun or rising moon.)

TO THE TRAILHEAD

GPS Coordinates: N32° 43.464181'   W117° 11.373117'
From I-5 just north of downtown San Diego, follow the signs for San Diego International Airport. Signs will direct you onto westbound North Harbor Drive. Stay in the leftmost lane (right lanes go into the airport), and turn left on Harbor Island Drive. Proceed 0.3 mile to where Harbor Island Drive splits east and west. Turn left (east) and drive to a spacious public parking lot at the end of the road, 0.5 mile ahead.

30 Mission Valley San Diego River Trail

Trailhead Location: Mission Valley in San Diego

Trail Use: Hiking, running, dog walking, biking, skating

Distance & Configuration: 3-mile out-and-back

Elevation Range: Slightly above sea level throughout

Facilities: Just off the route, you will find a cornucopia of shopping, dining, and lodging venues.

Highlights: A linear oasis of serenity in the busiest part of Mission Valley

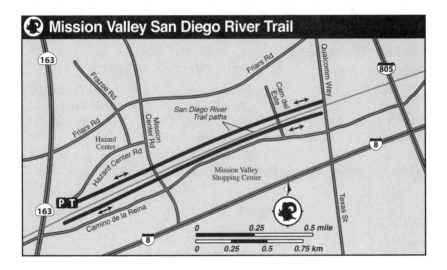

DESCRIPTION

Bounded by some 32 freeway lanes carrying more than a half million vehicles a day, and smack dab in San Diego County's busiest commercial zone, the San Diego River greenway in Mission Valley offers a surprising bit of tranquility. An agreeable, though thoroughly artificial, simulation of a riparian habitat exists here now, in stark contrast to the massive ripping apart of the landscape that took place in the early 1990s.

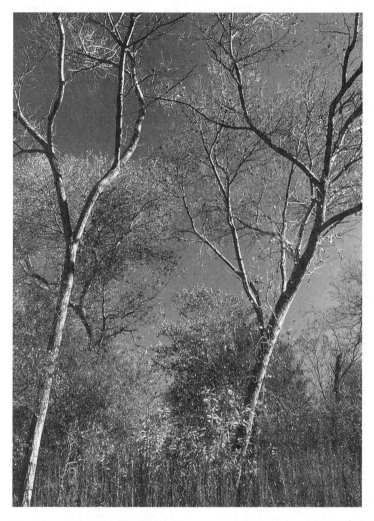

Riparian vegetation along the San Diego River

The First San Diego River Improvement Project, as the flood channel and greenway is known today, stretches between State Route 163 and
I-805. Designed for both flood control and wildlife habitat, the project has
so far contained the challenges of winter storm runoff and attracts its fair
share of resident and migrating waterfowl.

Wide concrete sidewalks follow both the north and the south banks
of the river between Qualcomm Way and a point west of Mission Village

Road near SR 163. The paths will likely be extended farther east and west along the river upon completion of future habitat-improvement projects. For nonmotorized travelers, a continuous path called the San Diego River Trail ultimately will be in place between the ocean at Ocean Beach and the headwaters of the San Diego River near the mountain community of Julian.

About 3 miles of walking, running, skating, or cycling suffices to cover the existing paths. The last decade has seen a remarkable growth of seeded riparian vegetation along the paths and along the riverbank. The now jungle-like screen of mature willow, sycamore, and cottonwood trees blots out the view of the river from most spots, so that bird-watching is possible only from a few select vantage points. The flora's rampant growth, however, is effective in diffusing the sounds of omnidirectional traffic and the occasional overhead passage of the San Diego Trolley on elevated tracks.

THE ROUTE

A good place to start this route, as noted on the map, is along Hazard Center Drive, just south of the Hazard Center shopping area. Just head south from there to pick up the north-riverbank sidewalk. Another possible starting point is on Camino de la Reina near Camino del Este or Qualcomm Way. Explore both the north-side and south-side paths, if you have the time.

During the early morning or after rush hour on a summer evening, the frenzy of mechanized transportation slackens, and you can hear the twittering of birds, the buzz of insects, and the whisper of leaves fluttering in the sea breeze. Your eyes may catch sight of butterflies and iridescent hummingbirds flitting among the flowers, and your nose will surely appreciate the sweet-pungent fragrance of the water-loving vegetation.

TO THE TRAILHEAD
GPS Coordinates: N32° 46.132257'   W117° 9.604318'
Exit SR 163 at Friars Road. Go east on Friars to the first major street (Frazee Road) and turn right. Go south to Hazard Center Drive, turn right, and find a parking space wherever you can.

31 Tecolote Canyon

Trailhead Location: East of Mission Bay

Trail Use: Hiking, dog walking, running, mountain biking

Distance & Configuration: Up to 5 miles out-and-back

Elevation Range: 50 feet at the start to 200 feet

Facilities: Water and restrooms at the start

Highlights: Pleasant springtime wildflowers and greenery

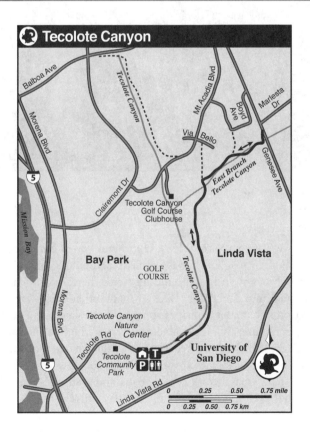

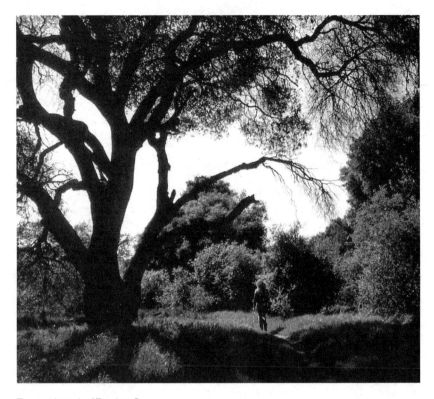

The east branch of Tecolote Canyon

DESCRIPTION

The 900-acre Tecolote Canyon Natural Park knifes into two of San Diego's older and denser suburban neighborhoods, namely Clairemont and Linda Vista. World War II brought an initial building frenzy here, and intensive development continued into the 1970s. Like so many other places around San Diego, the canyon floor and its hillsides appeared to be slated for a major roadway and still more houses, but local advocates turned the tide and saved the canyon. Today, Tecolote Canyon is regarded as a valued habitat for native plants and animals and also welcomes anyone curious enough to visit.

On the natural park's patchwork of old roads and trails, it's possible to poke into just about every nook and cranny. By day you're sure to spot a hawk soaring on the thermals or perching high on the crown of a dead oak tree. By night you might hear the yapping of a coyote or the plaintive hoot of an owl, the creature for which this canyon was named.

For all but the most cursory exploration of this canyon, you should wear hiking boots or at least a pair of running shoes designed for off-road traction. Parts of the trail system are rough, but even small kids will like it—though perhaps not if they are forced to go too far.

THE ROUTE

Only the lower two-thirds of Tecolote's trail system is covered on our map. In addition to the primary trailhead next to the Tecolote Canyon Nature Center, the park has eight other neighborhood trail access points, and some of those are north of Balboa Avenue.

Here, we concentrate on the main, wide, smooth path going up Tecolote Canyon's broad lower end. The first mile is fine for casual walking, jogging, and mountain biking, at least at first. You can look at the sage scrub and chaparral vegetation, at least in the late winter and spring when such plants are green and flowery. Down along the canyon's small stream channel, live oaks, willows, and sycamores thrive.

After about a mile, as you approach the perimeter of the Tecolote Canyon Golf Course, you'll start struggling up and down some steep hillsides. A narrow path on the left contours above the golf course, not far above the perimeter fence. It bends east on the slope overlooking the golf clubhouse and descends to an east branch of the canyon. The hike up along this fine, oak- and sycamore-dotted finger canyon to as far as Genesee Avenue is well worth it. If you reverse your steps upon reaching Genesee and return to the starting point, your round-trip hike measures about 5 miles.

TO THE TRAILHEAD

GPS Coordinates: N32° 46.540139'   W117° 11.841424'
Exit I-5 at SeaWorld Drive/Tecolote Road. Drive 0.6 mile east on Tecolote Road to reach Tecolote Community Park and the nature center for Tecolote Canyon Natural Park immediately beyond.

32 Bankers Hill

Trailhead Location: Just north of downtown San Diego

Trail Use: Hiking, dog walking, running

Distance & Configuration: 2.3-mile loop

Elevation Range: 80 feet at start to 290 feet in Bankers Hill

Facilities: One restaurant/store midway into the hike

Highlights: Historic houses and century-old footbridges

DESCRIPTION

With its quaint footbridges spanning two wooded ravines, scores of historic homes, plus a wealth of mature landscaping, Bankers Hill speaks to historical elegance and the preservation of nature. The following short ramble through canyon bottom and along quiet city streets takes you there—north and south, top and bottom.

THE ROUTE

From the end of Maple Street, make your way on foot up the wide, smooth path in the canyon bottom ahead, noting the mix of native sage scrub and chaparral vegetation and the nonnative eucalyptus trees and palm trees, the latter giving plenty of shade.

At about 100 yards into the canyon, notice the steep slope to the right. At the top, on the canyon rim, lies a historical marker commemorating the 1909 aviation feats of Waldo Waterman, who sailed off this perch on a homemade contraption and glided into the canyon bottom without breaking his neck. The plaque, up at the corner of Albatross and Maple, is better suited for a drive-by visit than a side trip climb on foot.

Farther up the canyon floor, you pass under the tall and graceful First Avenue Bridge, erected in 1912 and upgraded to modern engineering standards in 2009. After nearly 0.5 mile, you reach the wooden supporting beams of the equally historic Quince Street footbridge. A steep path through eucalyptus trees on the left, with log stairs, connects to Third Avenue and houses above. Trudge upward and make a right on Third Avenue.

After only a half block, turn left on Redwood Street, and continue two blocks to First Avenue. You're now squarely in the historic Bankers

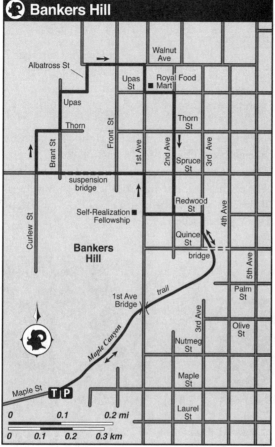

Hill neighborhood, where many of the city's elite resided a century ago. Once you reach First, gaze across the street to spot the Self-Realization Fellowship, formerly Bishop's Day School (1908), partially designed by San Diego's renowned architect Irving Gill. The Gill-designed wing wraps around an older Tudor structure and epitomizes Gill's philosophy of simplicity and, using his own phrase, "monastic severity."

From Redwood and First, continue north on First Avenue to Spruce Street. (In case you hadn't noticed, east-west streets are ordered alphabetically from Ash and Beech in downtown San Diego to Redwood and Spruce and beyond in Bankers Hill.) Make a left on Spruce Street and head west (downhill) to cross the 1912 Spruce Street suspension footbridge over a ravine commonly known as Arroyo Canyon. Pause in the middle of the swaying bridge, 70 feet above the canyon floor, and feel the breeze sweeping up-canyon from the bay.

On solid ground again at Brant Street, continue west another block to Curlew Street and turn right—all the while taking note of the varied architectural styles of the homes, most of which date back to the early 20th century. Many of the properties display historical plaques indicating the date of original construction.

Heading north on Curlew, you soon make a right on Thorn Street. Zigzag east on Thorn, north on Brant Street, east on Upas Street, and north on Albatross Street. On the east side of Albatross are some of Irving Gill's noted canyon houses, dating from 1912–13 and designed to blend harmoniously with the natural landscape of the ravine below. From Albatross, make a right on Walnut Street and proceed two blocks

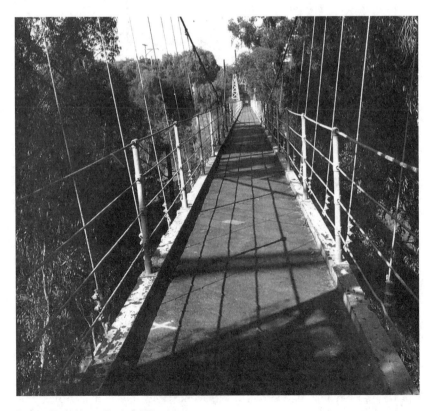

Suspension bridge at Bankers Hill

to First Avenue. Turn right and within a short block reach the Royal Food Mart, a restaurant housed in an early 1900s structure whose exterior appearance and interior furnishings are suggestive of that time in history. Take a break for food or beverages here if you like. Outside tables are available.

From the restaurant, go one block east on Upas Street to Second Avenue, and turn right. Enjoy the grand old homes in the next three blocks ahead. When you reach Redwood, go left for a block, turn right on Third, and finally make your descent into Maple Canyon, retracing your former route in the canyon bottom and back to your starting point.

TO THE TRAILHEAD

GPS Coordinates: N32° 43.933618'   W117° 10.053842'

Travel north on State Street out of downtown San Diego's Little Italy neighborhood to Laurel Street, where there is a traffic light. Continue one block north and turn right on Maple Street. There are actually multiple aligned and discontinuous segments of Maple Street stretching eastward for several miles, so make sure that you are on the correct one—just past that Laurel and State intersection. This segment of Maple Street ends two blocks east at a sign indicating MAPLE STREET OPEN SPACE PARK. Curbside parking is available.

33 Balboa Park's West Mesa

Trailhead Location: Northwest corner of Balboa Park

Trail Use: Hiking, running, dog walking, biking, wheelchair use

Distance & Configuration: 1.5-mile loop

Elevation Range: 250–300 feet

Facilities: Water and public restrooms available throughout; several restaurants on Fifth Avenue, one block west of the route

Highlights: Exquisitely landscaped parkland

DESCRIPTION

Balboa Park's historic buildings, museums, gardens, and the world-famous San Diego Zoo have pretty much framed the site's reputation for decades. What many visitors and even locals don't know is that Balboa sprawls over a total of 1,200 acres, or nearly 2 square miles. That's a lot of space to explore for the self-propelled traveler.

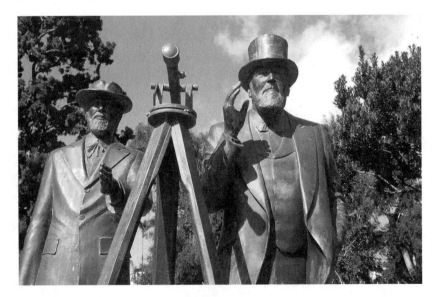

Horton and Marston statues

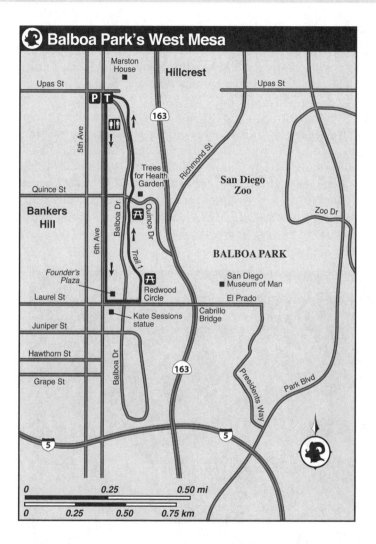

Incremental improvements have taken place over the past several years throughout Balboa Park's hidden spaces. Canyon slopes formerly choked with weedy undergrowth and once used as drug dens have been cleared out and made user-friendly and safer for local residents and tourists. Forgotten pathways have been reconstructed, and new landscaping has been installed. As part of this process, the park has established five trail gateways (trailheads) and numerous marked trail routes that serve every corner of the park.

THE ROUTE

Balboa Park's exquisitely landscaped West Mesa section along Sixth Avenue is the destination for the hike described here. You'll follow Trail 1, the shortest and smoothest (almost entirely sidewalk) of the five routes that emanate from the Sixth and Upas Gateway.

From the gateway sign at Sixth and Upas, head south on the palm-lined sidewalk along Sixth Avenue. At infrequent intervals, you see small trail signs guiding the way. The signage is innovative: Each sign has a background color—blue for Sixth and Upas trails and other colors for the other four gateways. The number for each trail lies inside a geometric outline (round for an easy trail, square for a medium difficulty trail, and diamond for a difficult trail). Signs have directional arrows and often have a cumulative mileage figure.

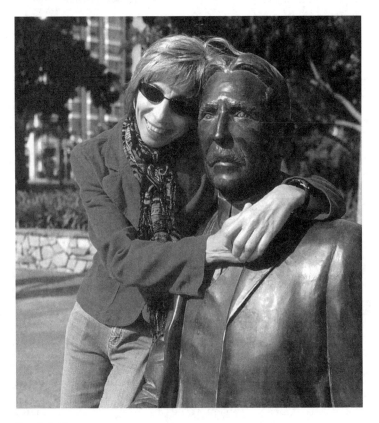

Founder's Plaza

After ten blocks of sidewalk travel, the Trail 1 sign directs you leftward on Laurel Street/El Prado, the street that crosses over the long Cabrillo Bridge to the east. As you make that turn, check out Founder's Plaza on the left, with lifelike statues of Balboa Park's early proponents. On the right, across El Prado, lies the statue of Kate Sessions, the horticulturist known as the mother of Balboa Park. Starting in 1892, Sessions planted thousands of trees from around the world on what was at that time dry, scrubby hilltops and hillsides. Today, the landscaping on West Mesa serves as a de facto botanical garden and arboretum.

Cross Balboa Drive, heading east toward the start of the Cabrillo Bridge (take the sidewalk across the bridge toward Balboa Park's historic section if you are so inclined for a side trip). The Trail 1 route, though, veers left just before the start of the bridge. You skirt a perfectly manicured lawn-bowling court and curve around a picnic site called Redwood Circle. Yes, those are coast redwoods planted around the periphery, far from their native foggy habitat up north. They do look a bit scraggly due to San Diego's sunny climate.

As you continue north, now and again you'll catch a treetop-level vista, off to the right, of the dominant building in the park's historic area: the Museum of Man's California Tower. Farther ahead lies a crossing of Quince Drive and a short passage through the Trees for Health Garden, which highlights medicinal native and nonnative plants and trees.

As you approach Upas Street, note a couple of gnarled oaks with puffy bark on the right. They're in fact cork oaks. Dig your fingernails into the soft bark to find out for sure. On a bit farther, just short of the historic Marston House (tours offered), you return to your starting point.

Trail 1 is barely an introduction to the West Mesa–centered trails. You may print out detailed, full-color maps of all five of the Sixth and Upas trails, plus other maps of Balboa Park, from **balboapark.org.**

TO THE TRAILHEAD
GPS Coordinates: N32° 44.444282'   W117° 9.556260'
From I-5 or from downtown San Diego, take State Route 163 north. Exit at the first ramp, Quince Drive. Quince takes you up to Sixth Avenue. Turn right on Sixth, go four blocks north to Upas Street, and find curbside parking on any street near the intersection of Sixth and Upas.

34 Balboa Park's Central Mesa

Trailhead Location: Central Balboa Park

Trail Use: Hiking, running, dog walking

Distance & Configuration: 3-mile loop

Elevation Range: 200–300 feet

Facilities: Water and public restrooms near the middle of the route

Highlights: Rose and succulent gardens, historic buildings and plazas, crossing the high Cabrillo Bridge

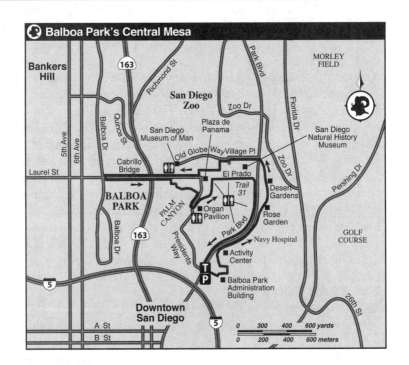

DESCRIPTION

Balboa Park's Central Mesa incorporates two historical sectors: the 1915–16 Panama-California Exposition site on the north and the 1935–36 California Pacific International Exposition site on the south. Both expositions were fielded by the then-relatively-small city of San Diego for the purpose of gaining international attention. As in the case of nearly all world's fairs, the theme buildings hastily constructed for both expositions found later uses, such as housing museums and a variety of civic and cultural organizations.

The 1915–16 exposition site in particular is renowned among San Diegans for its incomparably beautiful Spanish-Moorish buildings, its gardens, and the graceful Cabrillo Bridge. That area is therefore the primary destination of this short hike. You'll be following signs for Trail 31 throughout.

THE ROUTE

From the Park Boulevard Gateway sign, first head east on the sidewalk leading directly toward the Balboa Park administration building. Climb the stairs, swing left around the headquarters building, and enjoy the pergola-bounded courtyard behind it. Comparatively few people visit this beautiful space.

From the courtyard, walk north and edge by the Balboa Park Activity Center (table tennis, badminton, volleyball, and the like are practiced inside). You emerge along the sidewalk following Park Boulevard. Continue north along the fenced perimeter of the Navy Hospital. After a short distance you come upon the spacious Rose Garden and just past that, the Desert Gardens, a hillside covered with exotic succulent plants from around the world.

At the far north end of the Desert Gardens, you arrive at the intersection of Park Boulevard and Village Place. Cross Park Boulevard at the traffic light there, and head west past the massive Moreton Bay fig tree that stands in front of the entrance to the San Diego Natural History Museum.

At the next street crossing, jog slightly left and pick up Old Globe Way on the far side. You skirt the south boundary fence of the San Diego Zoo for a short while, and then turn left, just short of the open-lath Botanical Building. Bear right alongside the front entrance to the Botanical Building, passing right over the majestically serene Lily Pond. Need we say that you should have your camera along?

Just ahead, you reach the park's central square, Plaza de Panama, bounded by two art museums on the north and various historical structures dating from the 1915–16 exposition on the south. The plaza is now devoted to parked cars, but it's slated to be transformed into pedestrian-only gathering space in time for the exposition's centennial in 2015.

Following Trail 31 signs (which are plaques imbedded in the sidewalk within the park's historical zones), continue west along El Prado, past the Museum of Man's lofty California Tower, and all the way across the Cabrillo Bridge, using the north-side sidewalk. The 450-foot-long, 120-foot-high bridge, begun in 1912, uses a multiple-arched cantilever structure, which was innovative at that time and timeless in its form.

At the far side of the bridge, cross over the El Prado roadway and pick up the south-side sidewalk for the reverse direction (east). The historic Cabrillo Freeway (better known as the 163 freeway) curves below, leading toward the cluster of high-rises that defines San Diego's downtown skyline. Many a classic postcard photo was taken from this vantage.

Returning to the California Tower, veer right just ahead for a passage through Alcazar Gardens and edge along the lushly landscaped upper rim of Palm Canyon. You then curve left toward the Organ Pavilion, which houses one of the world's largest pipe organs. Travel north from there past the Japanese Friendship Garden, and return to Plaza de Panama.

Make a right now, and go east on the traffic-free section of El Prado, passing museums on both sides. Continue all the way to the circular fountain. Finally, make your way down to the west-side sidewalk on Park Boulevard, swing right, and follow that sidewalk back to the corner of Park Boulevard and Presidents Way, your starting point.

TO THE TRAILHEAD
GPS Coordinates: N32° 43.537438'   W117° 9.018838'
From downtown San Diego, follow Park Boulevard (12th Avenue) north. Right after passing over I-5, make a right at the first traffic light, Presidents Way. Park your car in one of the spacious lots near that intersection or along Park Boulevard itself. The Park Boulevard trail gateway sign is located at the northeast corner of Park Boulevard and Presidents Way.

35 Balboa Park's East Side

Trailhead Location: Just east of downtown San Diego

Trail Use: Hiking, dog walking, running

Distance & Configuration: 4.4-mile loop with spurs

Elevation Range: The route goes up and down several times, staying between 100 feet and 340 feet of elevation.

Facilities: Water and restrooms at the start and at Morley Field Sports Complex, midway through the hike

Highlights: Explore Balboa Park's far-east quarter, beautifully landscaped in places and home to several unsung attractions.

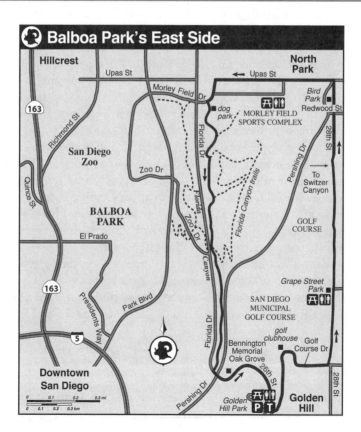

DESCRIPTION

Balboa Park's easternmost section isn't well known among most San Diegans, let alone tourists. Local residents, along with local golfers, do know of several out-of-the-way features here: Golden Hill Park, San Diego's Municipal Golf Course, Grape Street dog park, Switzer Canyon, and Bird Park. Exploring this spacious area is the goal of this hike, which follows Trail 22 in the Balboa Park trails system. You'll be on a combination of unpaved trails (some briefly steep and rocky), sidewalks, and roadside shoulders.

THE ROUTE

Starting from the Golden Hill Park trail gateway sign, head east and downhill from 25th Street to the four-way stop sign at 26th Street. Go straight across to Golf Course Drive, and stay on the left (west) wood-chip-surfaced shoulder of that two-lane road. Follow the road as it curves past the golf course clubhouse. Look behind to catch an unusual (if you haven't been in these parts before) vista of the downtown San Diego skyline.

Past a couple more curves, Golf Course Drive intersects with 28th Street. Very near that intersection, make a left on the signed trail heading due north. Due north you go, paying no heed to the topography, down one steep hill and up another slope to flat land again. You go by the Grape Street picnic area and dog park on the left, only one of three areas within Balboa Park where unleashed dogs can roam.

Continue following the north-heading Trail 22, losing elevation again. You find yourself right alongside one of the golf course's fairways, fringed with a beautiful grove of planted native live oaks. Just ahead you'll see an informational signboard for the Switzer Canyon open space, a small city-owned natural area occupying the canyon on the right side. Keep going straight, though, steeply uphill, and hook up with 28th Street on the rim of Switzer Canyon, staying to the right of the golf course.

Use the sidewalk of 28th Street to travel north for five blocks to Upas Street, passing numerous homes of historical importance. Notice the contractor's date stamps in the sidewalk concrete slabs. Bird Park, a mini-park within Balboa Park at 28th and Upas Streets, pays homage to San Diego's great variety of native birds.

Now head west on Upas Street for 0.5 mile, hang a left on Morley Field Drive, continue about 100 yards, and hang a left again at the entrance to a parking lot next to the Morley Field dog park. Travel south through the dog park and pick up the trail descending into Florida Canyon, Balboa

Park's primary area of native vegetation. Try to realize that at first glance the natural vegetation of Florida Canyon may appear scruffy and desiccated by comparison with the lushly (but artificially) landscaped acres of Balboa Park proper. The aesthetic differences between the two are minimized in late winter and early spring when new growth burgeons, the sage and other aromatic plants emit sweet fragrances, and wildflowers carpet the ground.

Keep heading south, on the left (east) side of Florida Drive and more or less parallel to it, for just over 1 mile. You then reach the intersection of Pershing Drive, Florida Drive, and 26th Street on the far side. Use the pedestrian crosswalks and walk signals to get across to 26th Street, a curving road leading upward. Follow the right shoulder of the road, which doubles as the final leg of Trail 22. On the lower half of this climb, take note of the beautiful grove of live oaks arching over you, called the Bennington Memorial Oak Grove. Its trees were planted in memory of the more than 60 men killed in the boiler steam explosion that took place aboard the USS *Bennington* gunboat in San Diego harbor in 1905.

TO THE TRAILHEAD

GPS Coordinates: N32° 43.210859'   W117° 8.458078'

From Broadway or Market Street, the two main east-west streets in downtown San Diego, travel east to 25th Street, turn left, and go north to where 25th Street ends at Golden Hill Park. Park for free in Golden Hill Park or on city streets. Look for the blue Balboa Park trail gateway signboard at the far north end of 25th Street.

36 San Diego Zoo

Trailhead Location: Balboa Park

Trail Use: Hiking

Distance & Configuration: 1.3-mile loop

Elevation Range: 150–250 feet

Facilities: All facilities along the route

Highlights: The thickest vegetation and the densest shade you can find in San Diego

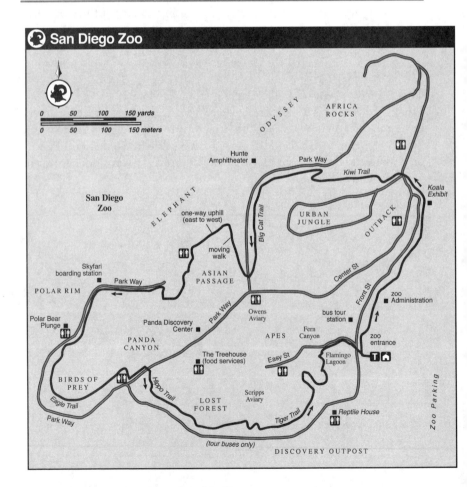

DESCRIPTION

For a bit of morning exercise, especially if you're a local San Diegan, consider this quick jaunt at the San Diego Zoo, not normally thought of as a hiking destination. Get there at opening time (9 a.m. daily) and you'll likely be the only person treading certain portions of the 1.3-mile looping route described here. On a typical day, 10 a.m. is too late. There will be too many gawking individuals and baby strollers to contend with on the narrow paths.

The route remains mostly out of the sun, under cover of exotic trees and junglelike vegetation as much as possible, so it's perfect for San Diego's warmer mornings, which tend to occur July–October. Oh yes, we should mention the fact that you might be tempted to linger at one exhibit or another, since 9 a.m. happens to be a perfect time to see the zoo animals up close—not hidden in the back of their enclosures. If exercise is your primary goal, then consider using the same route for two loops, or even three. The zoological scenery changes constantly.

Visitors who purchase a membership to the San Diego Zoological Society receive 365 days of free admission to both the San Diego Zoo and the San Diego Zoo Safari Park in Escondido. With a membership, you simply glide through the entrance gate with membership card and picture ID.

Once inside the zoo, pick up a color map (at the map rack to the right), which features far more detail than this page's sketch map includes. *Note that the zoo's color map is oriented west-up, not the standard north-up.*

THE ROUTE

Staying right, follow the sidewalk along Front Street. At about 0.2 mile you pass the Koala Exhibit on the right. Beyond the intersection of Front Street and Center Street, you arrive at the turnoff for the Urban Jungle section of the zoo. Cross Front Street there and pick up the signed Kiwi Trail, a narrow hardscape path that soon darts downward along a shady hillside. Just shy of Park Way, you make a hard left to stay on the narrow path, which is now called Big Cat Trail. Sure enough, you stroll right by jaguar, mountain lion, and leopard enclosures.

After about 0.5 mile of total travel, you dip to touch Park Way. Go across that street and pick up the one-way moving walk on the far side. Signs advise you to stay still, so at least savor the fact that you can gain some gravitational potential energy at no muscular expense. At the top, you emerge at the edge of the newest and most elaborate of the zoo's exhibits, Elephant Odyssey, which will sorely tempt you to engage in a side trip.

Keeping in mind the purpose of our 1.3-mile focused march, press on south and join Park Way. Stroll past the Skyfari (chair-lift) station and the Polar Bear Plunge exhibit, and curve left past the Birds of Prey exhibit, using the Eagle Trail.

After descending to Park Way, follow the left-side sidewalk for about 100 feet, and then swing right (going across Park Way) to pick up the Hippo Trail. You've come about a mile so far and have only a third of a mile to go, albeit an almost entirely uphill segment, to complete the loop.

Past the hippos, take care to stay right on the Tiger Trail, which will take you through the deepest, darkest part of the zoo landscape (not to mention past a host of interesting captive animals).

When you reach a point where you are almost directly underneath a steel bridge, swing right to remain on Tiger Trail. After a bit more climbing, you emerge on sunny Easy Street. Swing right, and complete the last few steps to where you began your journey.

TO THE TRAILHEAD

GPS Coordinates: N32° 44.115121'   W117° 8.965738'

From downtown San Diego, drive north on Park Boulevard (12th Avenue) for about 1 mile. Turn left at Zoo Place, and enter the San Diego Zoo parking lot (free parking).

37 The Embarcadero

Trailhead Location: Downtown San Diego

Trail Use: Hiking, running, dog walking, bicycling

Distance & Configuration: 3-mile out-and-back with a loop

Elevation Range: Sea level throughout

Facilities: Everywhere along the route

Highlights: Bay and city vistas from San Diego's front porch

DESCRIPTION

San Diego's Embarcadero, the place of departure and arrival for vessels as small as fishing skiffs and as large as ocean liners, defines the city's connection to the watery worlds of San Diego Bay and the Pacific Ocean. The unquestionably spectacular views of today are somewhat marred by a preponderance of all-too-wide thoroughfares given over to car traffic, parking lots, and hulking military buildings dating from decades ago.

All that is changing and will evolve over the next decade or more as several major redevelopment projects come online to spiff up the waterfront with wide walkways, grassy parks for picnics and entertainment events, more restaurants and retail outlets, and a remade skyline immediately inland. That means that our directions for travel along the Embarcadero will remain somewhat tentative for years to come.

THE ROUTE

A good starting place is the winding concrete sidewalk that follows the bay shoreline just north of the traffic lights at North Harbor Drive and Hawthorn and Grape streets. There you'll find the northernmost of the 30 or so *Urban Trees* monumental sculptures that seemingly grow out of outsize flowerpots. The *Urban Trees* exhibit, sponsored by the Port of San Diego, is updated on a more or less yearly basis, with many of the older sculptures finding new homes on public and private properties all around San Diego. *Urban Trees* line the Embarcadero to as far as the Broadway Pier or beyond.

As you stroll south, the sidewalk widens, and you pass the collection of antique watercraft comprising the Maritime Museum of San Diego. The museum's signature attraction, the 1863 iron-hulled sailing vessel *Star of*

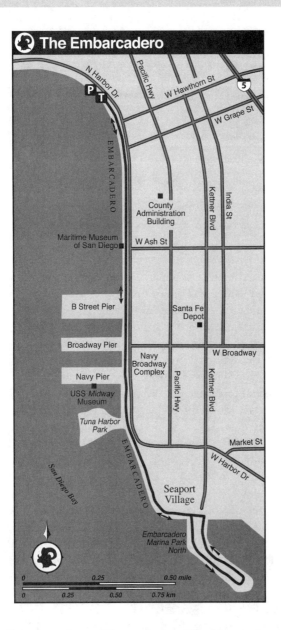

The Embarcadero

N Harbor Dr

Pacific Hwy

W Hawthorn St

W Grape St

5

P T

EMBARCADERO

County
Administration
Building

Kettner Blvd

India St

Maritime Museum
of San Diego

W Ash St

B Street Pier

Santa Fe
Depot

Broadway Pier

Navy
Broadway
Complex

W Broadway

Navy Pier

Pacific Hwy

Kettner Blvd

USS *Midway*
Museum

Tuna Harbor
Park

EMBARCADERO

Market St

W Harbor Dr

San Diego Bay

Seaport
Village

Embarcadero
Marina Park
North

0   0.25   0.50 mile

0   0.25   0.50   0.75 km

India, currently qualifies as the world's oldest active ship. Occasionally she can be seen tooling around San Diego Bay.

Next, on the bay side, are three major piers. The B Street Pier for cruise ships allows no pedestrian access. The Broadway Pier, an auxiliary terminal

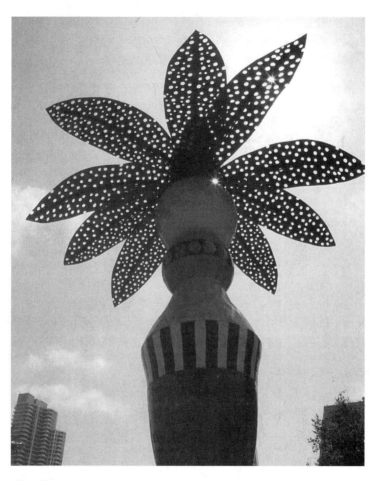

Urban Tree

for cruise ships, allows pedestrians when ships aren't docked there. Navy Pier, the southernmost of the three, has found a new use as a parking lot for the USS *Midway* aircraft carrier (now a museum), which is permanently berthed there. Small docks on either side of the Broadway Pier host vessels carrying tourists on bay excursions and whale-watching expeditions.

After Navy Pier, the sidewalk promenade widens to include Tuna Harbor Park. If you are inclined, take a short side trip over to various public art exhibits with World War II themes and to a viewpoint where you can look straight west toward the modern aircraft carriers at anchor alongside the North Island Naval Station. On the southwest side of Tuna Harbor Park lies a slightly gritty pier for commercial fishing boats. Walk out there to get a flavor for the San Diego working waterfront, complete with nets being repaired by commercial fishermen and lobster traps.

Resuming your travel south, you're quickly immersed in tourist heaven, with the shops and restaurants of Seaport Village on the left and a whitewashed smooth wall on the right, where you can sit and contemplate the whole of San Diego Bay's south arm, flecked with sailboats on windy days. The graceful arch of the San Diego–Coronado Bridge vaults over the scene.

Make a fitting far end to your Embarcadero hike by following the looping sidewalk around the north section of Embarcadero Marina Park, just south of Seaport Village. The 360-degree vista from this grassy space encompasses the bay, a small-boat harbor jammed with pleasure craft, swanky hotels, and the nautically themed San Diego Convention Center.

When you return to Seaport Village, simply retrace your earlier steps, with the exception of any earlier side trips, back to your starting point.

TO THE TRAILHEAD

GPS Coordinates: N32° 43.528082'   W117° 10.436583'

On North Harbor Drive, fronting San Diego Bay, and as close to West Hawthorn Street as possible, find any metered parking place or pay parking lot. This area is the recommended starting point because parking tends to be more available.

38 Gaslamp Quarter

Trailhead Location: Downtown San Diego

Trail Use: Hiking

Distance & Configuration: 1-mile loop

Elevation Range: Near sea level throughout

Facilities: Water, restrooms, dining, and shopping are plentiful along the route.

Highlights: San Diego's best historical scenery by day and the city's most vibrant nightlife

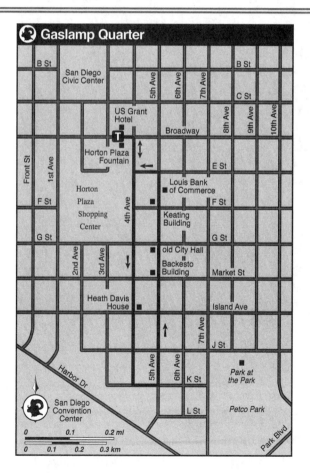

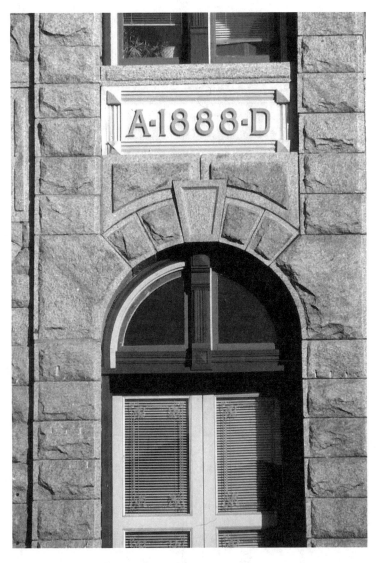

Historic building in the Gaslamp Quarter

DESCRIPTION

Formerly San Diego's skid row, this core downtown historic area was reborn in the 1980s under a new name: the Gaslamp Quarter. Actually, gas lamps were never used for outdoor lighting in San Diego, though today you can find a few decorative ones. Rather, the district's distinctive gas lamp–style electric streetlights pretty much inform you whether you're in the Gaslamp Quarter or not. This is the place to go in the daytime for scoping out dozens of historic buildings dating from the late 1800s through the early 1900s and (by night especially) for feeling the pulse of thousands of visitors milling about, drinking at watering holes, and dining in fine restaurants.

Ignoring small exceptions, the Gaslamp Quarter district stretches two blocks from west to east (Fourth and Sixth avenues) and eight blocks from north to south (Broadway to Harbor Drive). The cheek-by-jowl pattern of buildings in the Gaslamp is unique among all San Diego neighborhoods. The frontages range from a narrow 25 feet to a broad 225 feet. The latter is the case for one historic site, the 1873 Backesto Building on Fifth Avenue. You'll see modern (21st-century) architecture, but even that was designed to fit in harmoniously with the earlier structures.

THE ROUTE

A definitive starting point for our Gaslamp Quarter tour is the historic Horton Plaza fountain at Fourth Avenue and Broadway. The century-old fountain (which may be within the boundary of a construction zone for a new public plaza by 2014) was one of the first to combine colored lighting effects with flowing water. Across Broadway lies the elegant US Grant Hotel, dating from 1910.

Head south on Fourth Avenue, staying on the left (or east) side to remain close to a long row of historic buildings. More than 90 buildings throughout the Gaslamp are tagged with brass plaques, each including a short historical description. At the end of the fifth block (Fourth and Island Avenue), on the left, pay a visit to the William Heath Davis House (1850), the location of the Gaslamp Quarter Historical Foundation's visitor center. There you can pick up a guide map for the historic buildings in the Gaslamp district.

After traveling two more blocks south (nearly as far as Harbor Drive and the Convention Center), swing left on K Street and left again on Fifth Avenue. Now, as you head north on either side of Fifth, you're going to encounter the very best in historic architecture, or the wildest nightlife, assuming you're here during the late-night hours. Notable daytime sights include the old San Diego City Hall building (1874) at Fifth Avenue and G Street, the Backesto Building (the long, low one) at Fifth and Market Street, the 1890 Keating Building at Fifth and F Street, and the ornate 1888 Louis Bank of Commerce building on Fifth between E and F streets. When you reach E Street, head back to Fourth to return to Horton Plaza.

Naturally, you'll be tempted to stray off of the route described above. You can head west to check out San Diego's tiny Asian district centered at Third and Island, head south to follow the arrow-straight path through the Martin Luther King Jr. linear park paralleling Harbor Drive, or skip a few blocks east and picnic at the grassy Park at the Park, which is adjacent to the Petco Park baseball stadium.

TO THE TRAILHEAD

GPS Coordinates: N32° 42.935278'   W117° 9.691801'

Drive to the Horton Plaza shopping center bounded by Broadway, Fourth Avenue, G Street, and First Avenue in downtown San Diego. Park in the parking garage of the shopping center (up to 3 hours validated free parking). Or try to find a parking space (free on Sundays) along any downtown street or in any pay parking lot near Horton Plaza. Start your walk at the historic Horton Plaza fountain on Broadway at Fourth Avenue.

39 Coronado Beach

Trailhead Location: Coronado

Trail Use: Hiking, running, dog walking, night hiking

Distance & Configuration: 3.2-mile out-and-back

Elevation Range: Sea level all the way

Facilities: Access to water and public restrooms near the middle of the beach; Coronado's commercial district lies a few blocks east

Highlights: An extraordinarily wide beach, packed with fine-grained sand, and with a glorious view of Point Loma and the ocean

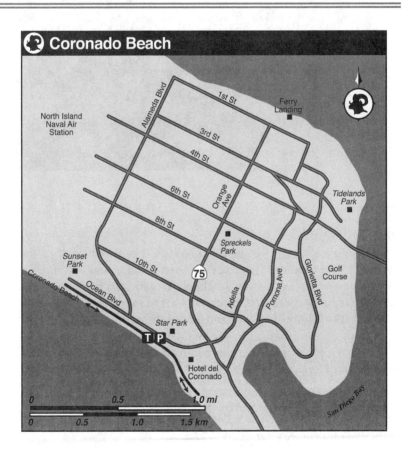

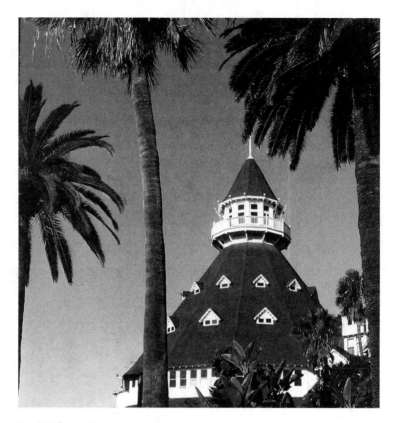

Hotel del Coronado

DESCRIPTION

Travel magazines routinely rank Coronado's oceanfront beach as one of the nation's most beautiful stretches of coastline, and you will surely agree with this assessment when you get there. Actually, the beach itself extends into military zones both to the north and to the south, and those areas have been strictly off-limits to public entry since the events of 9/11.

But the 1.6-mile stretch in the middle runs from North Beach in the north—or Dog Beach, where pets can roam free and swim—to the south edge of the Coronado Shores high-rise condominium development. In between lies the venerable Hotel del Coronado, affectionately known as the Hotel Del or The Del. Classified as a National Historic Landmark, the hotel first opened its doors in 1888 and was the setting for the shenanigans of the 1959 hit comedy *Some Like It Hot*.

Walking, wading, running, and swimming, not to mention building sand castles, are all popular pursuits here. (Note that pets are allowed only on the northernmost stretch.)

Why is the beach so wide? You'll get a hint when you look at the westward-pointing finger of the Point Loma peninsula. The prevailing California current sweeps south past the point, and some of the flow swirls east and north, depositing sand and sediment along a narrow sandbar called the Silver Strand, just south of Coronado. Plenty of that sand ends up on the shoreline of Coronado itself.

It's especially interesting to walk here during low tide, when the gently shelving wet sand extends far out to sea. Right in front of the hotel, at low tide only, some large rocks intentionally placed there to prevent erosion are exposed. During the lowest tides, some marine life, such as anemones, can be seen clinging to this artificial reef.

THE ROUTE

From wherever you score a parking spot, cross Ocean Boulevard and head across the side beach to the shoreline. (*Note:* At midday, that stretch of dry sand could be fiery hot, so bring at least a pair of flip-flops.) Turn either up-coast or down-coast and make the round-trip. Out-and-back for both segments, combined, totals 3.2 miles.

For a really memorable experience, time your visit on a late summer evening when there is a full moon. Plan to be wading north of the Hotel Del at sunset. Can you imagine 70°F water tickling your toes, while at the same time, a big yellow moon launches itself over the fairy-tale turrets of the hotel right in front of you?

TO THE TRAILHEAD

GPS Coordinates: N32° 40.955222'   W117° 10.959778'

From San Diego, take the toll-free San Diego–Coronado Bridge across San Diego Bay and into Coronado. The westbound lanes become Third Street. After several blocks on Third Street, turn left at the Orange Avenue traffic light. After 1 mile and as you approach the mammoth Victorian-style Hotel del Coronado, turn right on any street beyond Tenth Street. They all lead directly or indirectly west to Ocean Boulevard, which runs along the beach. Park on Ocean Boulevard or on any residential street just inland. At this point you'll be roughly in the middle of the publicly accessible stretch of Coronado Beach. This is the area where you will most likely find a parking space.

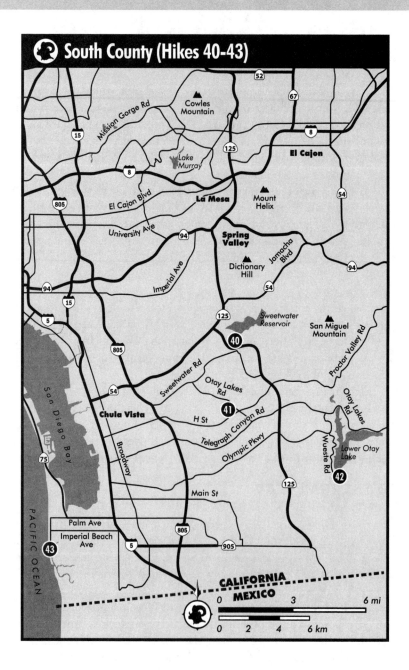
South County (Hikes 40-43)

SOUTH COUNTY

Regional Overview

South County, or the South Bay region as it is often called, spreads inland some 10 miles from the shores of South San Diego Bay. Chock-full of housing and industrial developments near the bay shore, the region gradually assumes a suburban and, finally, a semirural character as you travel east. Beyond the housing developments, rounded peaks and mountain ranges rise from rolling hills and broad valleys. Much of this currently empty zone is slated to fill up with residences accommodating much of San Diego County's future population growth.

The four hikes in this section have been chosen for ease of access. All feature well-defined trailheads. Parking (with the possible exclusion of hike 43, Imperial Beach, in the summer) is not a problem. Warm and dry midsummer days on routes such as hike 40, the Sweetwater Trail, warrant an early start or an extra-large water bottle. Otherwise, these South County hikes are short or easy and carefree.

◻ ◻ ◻

40 Sweetwater Trail

Trailhead Location: Bonita

Trail Use: Hiking, dog walking, running, mountain biking, horse-back riding

Distance & Configuration: 4.8-mile out-and-back

Elevation Range: 260 feet at the start to 480 feet at end

Facilities: Water and restrooms at the start

Highlights: Panoramic views of South San Diego County's mountain and foothill communities

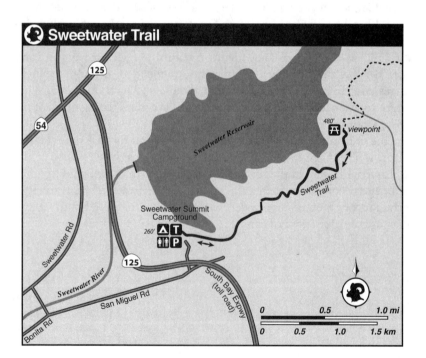

DESCRIPTION

San Diego's South Bay region—the coastal plain and foothills inland from South San Diego Bay—mixes up square miles worth of recently built housing tracts with pristine meadows and mountain slopes, albeit treeless ones. You can still find wide-open spaces where wild oats and foxtails chafe in the afternoon breeze, the spicy aroma of sage scents the air, hawks glide overhead, and coyotes and other small animals flourish.

One such space surrounds Sweetwater Reservoir in the semirural community of Bonita. Long before any significant modern settlement of the area, the Sweetwater Dam was built to impound the rather meager flow of runoff from mountains to the east and dole it out to agricultural lands during the summer dry season. At the time of its completion in 1888, the dam was higher than any other in the United States. Today, the dam and reservoir are merely bantam class, but they're a lovely addition to the landscape nonetheless.

Sensuously rounded hills—dotted with sage, pepper trees, and rare coastal varieties of cholla and barrel cactus—spread to the south and east of Sweetwater Reservoir. Running-shoe footprints overlap the linear marks of mountain-bike tires and the inverted-U impressions of horseshoes on the Sweetwater Trail that skirts the shore of the reservoir.

THE ROUTE

You pick up the best section of the Sweetwater Trail at the north end of Sweetwater Summit Campground. You head east, first passing a fishing access area for the reservoir and then traversing near-flat grassland. It's hot in the middle of the day, perhaps, but it's pleasant in early morning or late afternoon.

After about 1 mile, the trail veers sharply right and begins a series of relentless and rather severe ups and downs. You're aiming for the flat top of a prominent knoll ahead, where you'll find a picnic table under a shade ramada and a commanding view of the lake and much of the South Bay area. In the opposite direction rises the massive, triangular bulk of San Miguel Mountain, its summit bewhiskered by several spiky radio and TV broadcast antennas.

This fine view spot, 2.4 miles into the hike, is a good place to turn around. It is the termination point for this 4.8-mile route.

If you want to keep going, some additional 2 miles of hiking will get you to the foot of San Miguel Mountain. Beyond that, it is possible to follow trails and dirt paths paralleling the Sweetwater River all the way to State Route 94 at Rancho San Diego. Be forewarned that the right-of-way for this extension of the trail is not yet settled, so you may run into navigational problems if you choose to press on.

TO THE TRAILHEAD

GPS Coordinates: N32° 41.030939'   W117° 0.155640'

Exit I-805 at Bonita Road and go east for about 4 miles. Keep going straight on San Miguel Road at the intersection where Bonita Road swings abruptly north and crosses the Sweetwater River. After 1-plus mile on San Miguel Road, turn left on Summit Meadow Road, which leads to the north end of Sweetwater Summit Campground, the starting point for the hike. (*Note:* There is no access to San Miguel Road from the SR 125 toll road that passes over it.)

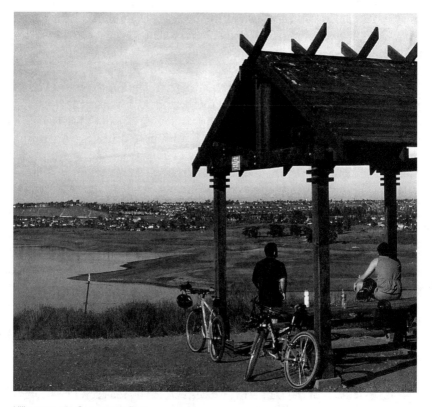

Hilltop ramada, Sweetwater Trail

41 Rice Canyon

Trailhead Location: Chula Vista

Trail Use: Hiking, dog walking, mountain biking, running

Distance & Configuration: 4-mile out-and-back

Elevation Range: 360 feet to 180 feet

Facilities: Water and public restrooms at Discovery Park, near the trailhead

Highlights: Easy strolling along a still-natural patch of canyon landscape

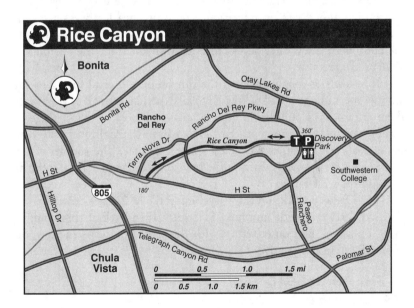

DESCRIPTION

On the scrub-covered slopes of Rice Canyon, hardy coast cholla cacti raise their asymmetric arms in what seems a gesture of defiance against the surrounding phalanxes of cookie-cutter, pseudo-Spanish-style homes. What remains of the formerly obscure and totally rural Rice Canyon has been incorporated into the city of Chula Vista's Rice Canyon Open Space

Preserve. There's a fine, wide trail following it for 2 miles, down to as far as H Street, 1 mile east of I-805.

Spring is by far the best time to enjoy the sights and fragrances of the canyon's plant life, most of which is classified as native riparian and coastal sage scrub. At the trailhead itself or at a mailbox about midway down the trail, a free leaflet produced by nearby Southwestern College may be available. If so, grab a copy, as its color photos and illustrations describe the canyon's native vegetation. You will learn interesting facts, such as that the largest bushes in sight on the canyon slopes are lemonade berry shrubs. Native Americans once used the shrubs' sticky fruit to prepare a beverage similar to lemonade.

THE ROUTE

From the sidewalk on the west side of Rancho Del Rey Parkway, across from Discovery Park, start heading west on the wide Rice Canyon Trail. Continuing along, you'll pass various side trails, nearly always associated with power line roads or other utility easements that run through the neighborhood. They offer access to Rice Canyon from the surrounding residential streets.

As you make your way down the canyon on a typical spring or early summer morning, you will be treated to an experience for all of your senses: The marine-layer clouds begin to part, and you'll breathe in salt-tinged air that pushes inland from south San Diego Bay. The California sagebrush plants coating the canyons exude a spicy fragrance. The sounds of bird, cricket, and cicada songs waft on the breeze. White and yellow butterflies flit amid the wildflowers.

Go as far as you like on this easygoing trail. At 2 miles down from the start, you arrive at wide and busy H Street. Turn back at this point and enjoy a peaceful and quiet return with the same landscape in view, only from a different perspective.

TO THE TRAILHEAD

GPS Coordinates: N32° 38.685'   W117° 0.677'

Exit I-805 at H Street in Chula Vista. Drive 2.8 miles east to Paseo Ranchero and turn left (north). Go 0.2 mile north to Rancho Del Rey Parkway. Turn right (east) and drive 0.3 mile to the Rice Canyon Trailhead on the left, opposite Discovery Park.

42 Lower Otay County Park

Trailhead Location: Eastern Chula Vista

Trail Use: Hiking, dog walking

Distance & Configuration: 0.8-mile out-and-back

Elevation Range: 520 feet at the start to 820 feet

Facilities: Water and restrooms at the start

Highlights: Spectacular vista of Lower Otay Reservoir to the north, mountains to the east, and suburbs to the west

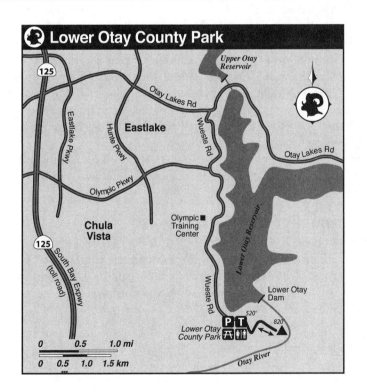

DESCRIPTION

Lower Otay County Park, on a hillside above the dam of Lower Otay Reservoir, was once a remote destination for most San Diegans. Now, due to the recent eastward spread of suburban development, the park lies within only a few minutes' drive for tens of thousands of South Bay residents. Not only that, but a recent renovation of the entire park has also turned it into a scenic spot for picnicking, with a fine view south into Mexico. To see farther, this hike engages you to make a short, steep climb to a hilltop.

THE ROUTE

From the topmost parking lot inside Lower Otay County Park, walk past a gate and go uphill on either an unpaved service road or on a parallel, zigzagging foot trail. Either way, you soon arrive at a resting bench offering an expansive view. Continue on the eroded firebreak that runs straight up the slope. You'll end up on a rounded knoll, high enough for you to see the Pacific Ocean, the terrestrial ocean of rooftops covering eastern Chula Vista, and—when clear enough—the upper floors of downtown San Diego's skyscrapers.

For the most impressive vista, however, gaze north toward Lower Otay Reservoir, which spreads its waters far and wide, seemingly at your feet. To the east, the long ridge of Otay Mountain climbs steadily toward the 3,572-foot high point of that range. This upward pitch, however, is interrupted by the Otay River gorge immediately below you, so the rounded summit is as far as you can conveniently go.

You've traveled a total of 0.4 mile to reach this scenic knoll and gained a quick 300 feet of elevation too. When it's time to return, simply retrace your steps.

TO THE TRAILHEAD

GPS Coordinates: N32° 36.454260'   W116° 55.745101'
Exit the SR 125 toll road at Olympic Parkway in east Chula Vista. Drive 2.7 miles east to Wueste Road and turn right (south). Continue south to the end of the road, where you'll find the entrance to Lower Otay County Park.

43 Imperial Beach

Trailhead Location: Imperial Beach

Trail Use: Hiking, dog walking

Distance & Configuration: 1.6-mile loop

Elevation Range: Sea level throughout

Facilities: Nearest water and restrooms 1 mile north at Imperial Beach Pier

Highlights: A rare, undeveloped stretch of beach facing the Pacific Ocean; abundant birdlife

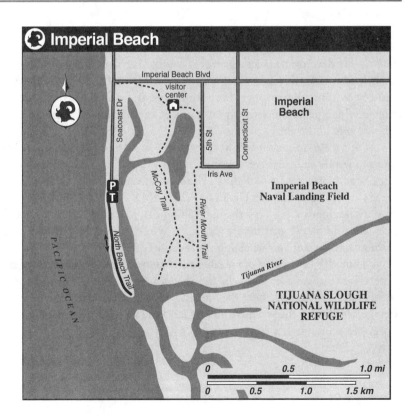

DESCRIPTION

At the south end of Seacoast Drive, a planked walkway and interpretive plaques introduce you to the green tidal marshlands of the Tijuana River Estuary to the east. The marshlands are part of a 4-square-mile tideland expanse managed by various national, state, and local agencies. This is one of Southern California's most important coastal wetland areas simply because it has been mostly spared from commercial and housing developments. The area is a recognized haven for birds, and more than 400 species have been logged here so far. This is no surprise because the estuary is a key stopover on the Pacific Flyway—the equivalent of I-5 for bird-migration traffic. The marsh's endangered inhabitants include the light-footed clapper rail and the California least tern. Visiting birds include ospreys, golden eagles, and peregrine falcons.

THE ROUTE

The walk itself begins with a little hop over rocks to the sandy beach. Modern houses and condominiums line the sandy strip to the north, but that's it for development as you travel south. Artificial dunes, off-limits to protect nesting terns, back up the beach to the left. At high tide, you could be edging close alongside those dunes, but low tide allows you to enjoy a wide, glassy-smooth expanse of wet sand, dimpled with rounded pebbles here and there.

At 0.8 mile from the start, you reach the mouth of the Tijuana River. Pause to appreciate this river's work: One-third of its drainage area covers San Diego County, and two-thirds drains a substantial part of Baja California (including the city of Tijuana). When storm runoff courses down the river, it's fascinating to watch the outrushing turbid freshwater mixing with the incoming blue-green ocean waves. In winter, gulls set up shop here, feeding in the water and wheeling overhead in great flocks.

Tijuana River water is of variable and often dubious quality, so it's not a great idea to wade or swim in the river's mouth. Most swimmers and surfers tend to hang out near the Imperial Beach Pier, where the beach is lifeguarded during the warmer months, and the water quality is better.

After some quality time river-gazing, return to your parked car the way you came.

TO THE TRAILHEAD

GPS Coordinates: N32° 33.993781'   W117° 7.936678'

Exit I-5 at Coronado Avenue in south San Diego. Turn west. Coronado Avenue becomes Imperial Beach Boulevard as you enter the city of Imperial Beach. Continue to the end of Imperial Beach Boulevard, and turn left (south) at Seacoast Drive. Public parking spaces line both sides of Seacoast Drive, which dead-ends 0.7 mile south. Find a space as close to the end as possible to position yourself at the beginning of your walk.

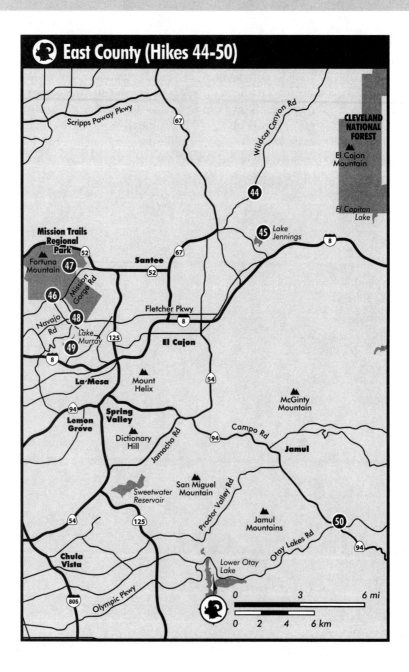

East County (Hikes 44-50)

Scripps Poway Pkwy

67

Wildcat Canyon Rd

CLEVELAND
NATIONAL
FOREST
El Cajon
Mountain

44

El Capitan
Lake

Mission Trails
Regional
Park

45   Lake
Jennings

8

52

Fortuna
Mountain   47

Santee

67

52

Mission Gorge Rd

46

Fletcher Pkwy

8

Navajo
Rd   48

El Cajon

Lake
Murray   49   125

La Mesa

Mount
Helix

54

McGinty
Mountain

94

Spring
Valley

Lemon
Grove

Dictionary
Hill

Jamacha Rd

Campo Rd

94

Jamul

San Miguel
Mountain

Sweetwater
Reservoir

Proctor Valley Rd

Jamul
Mountains

50

54

125

94

Chula
Vista

Lower Otay
Lake

Otay Lakes Rd

805

Olympic Pkwy

0   3   6 mi

0   2   4   6 km

EAST COUNTY

Regional Overview

What's commonly known among San Diegans as East County spreads inland from the easternmost city limits of San Diego. East County's westside communities—Santee, La Mesa, Lakeside, El Cajon, and Rancho San Diego—are effectively an extension of San Diego's inner-city suburbs.

Ten to 15 miles eastward, however, only the small communities of Alpine and Jamul, plus scattered rural properties, interrupt the generally wild character of the landscape. Several rocky promontories, such as El Cajon Mountain and Lyons Peak, rise to elevations of 3,000–4,000 feet.

Parks, preserves, and public open-space areas of all sizes are abundant in East County. The flagship Mission Trails Regional Park (at 6,000 acres now and soon to be expanded) sits right on the edge of the suburbs, which nearly surround it. Still, it is touted as one of the largest urban parks in the nation. Four of the seven hikes in this section lie inside the borders of Mission Trails Regional Park.

The other three hikes are a little more remote, but none typically will have you driving more than 30 minutes from downtown San Diego (traffic allowing). Again, as we've seen in earlier sections, these interior hikes are far better experienced in months outside the July–October hot, dry season.

◘ ◘ ◘

44 Louis Stelzer County Park

Trailhead Location: North of Lakeside

Trail Use: Hiking, running

Distance & Configuration: 3.6-mile loop, including two spurs

Elevation Range: 800 feet at the start to 1,372 feet at Stelzer Summit

Facilities: Water and restrooms at the trailhead

Highlights: Shade-giving oaks, as well as mountain and valley vistas

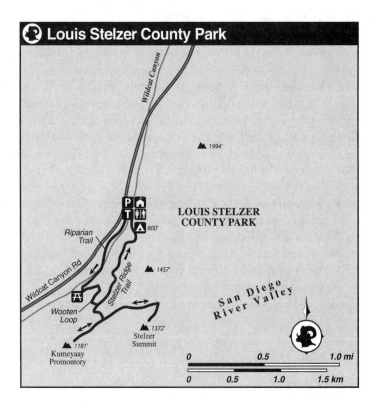

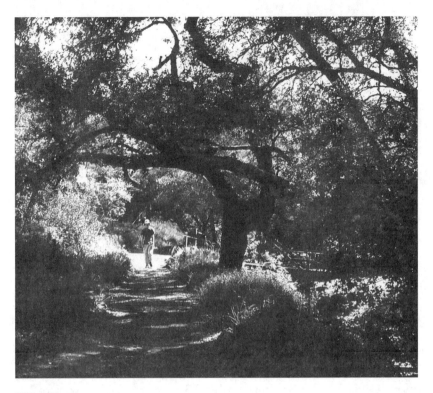

Wildcat Canyon

DESCRIPTION

The Louis Stelzer County Park, known simply as Stelzer Park, is operated by the County of San Diego Parks and Recreation. It devotes 314 acres to trails. A core area of campsites, picnic tables, and a small interpretive center nestle in the shady bottom of a steep ravine known as Wildcat Canyon. That area, next to the parking lot, was designed to accommodate persons with disabilities, though all visitors and hikers are welcome.

THE ROUTE

From the parking lot, start off by going south, parallel to Wildcat Canyon Road on the gradually descending Riparian Trail. The trail sticks closely to the stream bottom of Wildcat Canyon. As such it is semi-shaded by a stream-hugging canopy of live oaks, some draped with filigrees of wild-grape and poison-oak vines. The mammoth 2003 Cedar Fire swept through these oaks and into the upper-elevation slopes in this park, but most of the trees have survived more or less intact.

After 0.7 mile, the Riparian Trail ends at a secluded picnic site. From there, find and follow the trail marked Wooten Loop, which rises sharply on a slope to the east. After 0.3 mile of climbing, you reach Stelzer Ridge Trail. Hang a right and continue uphill to a wider trail on the ridgeline overlooking Wildcat Canyon.

Once there, for a better view, go 0.3 mile to the right to reach 1,181-foot Kumeyaay Promontory. Or go 0.4 mile to the left, up a very steep pitch, toward 1,372-foot Stelzer Summit. At Stelzer Summit, see if you can locate a rock pile atop the nearby hill. There, you will discover a hidden boulder-cave with an opening that overlooks a rural stretch of the San Diego River Valley. When the sea breeze blows up the valley, this becomes surely the coolest spot within the park. Off in the distance, down the valley, the bedroom communities of Lakeside and Santee spread coastward.

When you are through with the side trips, return to the junction of Stelzer Ridge and Wooten Loop. Follow the easily descending Stelzer Ridge Trail back to the park's core area and your starting point.

TO THE TRAILHEAD
GPS Coordinates: N32° 53.263800'   W116° 53.526778'
From Lakeside, where the SR 67 freeway segment ends at a traffic light, turn east on Mapleview Street. After 0.3 mile on Mapleview, turn left (north) on Ashwood Street. Ashwood will become Wildcat Canyon Road ahead. From the beginning of Ashwood, proceed 2 miles to Stelzer Park on the right. The trailhead parking lot is immediately past the park's entrance, where you can pay the small fee.

45 Lake Jennings

Trailhead Location: Lakeside

Trail Use: Hiking, mountain biking, running

Distance & Configuration: 1.6-mile out-and-back

Elevation Range: 750 feet at the start to 775 feet at the viewpoint

Facilities: No facilities along the trail; water, restrooms, and bait shop near the lake's entrance

Highlights: Extraordinary springtime color

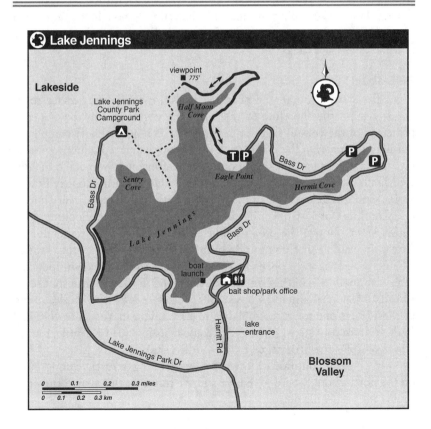

DESCRIPTION

Your impression of Lake Jennings may be strongly colored by the season in which you choose to visit. This is true for many of San Diego County's inland, low-elevation locales. Summer's heat and drought bleach all vibrant color from the vegetation, so that by July—and through the first rainstorms late in the year—the only color you see besides beige and brown is the blue of the sky and of Lake Jennings itself. In most years, though, February–April brings an almost unbelievable wave of green to the hillsides surrounding the lake. Also, in wetter years the profusion of wildflowers can be astounding.

Lake Jennings stores mostly imported water that when filtered becomes drinking water for more than a quarter million people in the East County region. For local residents, the lake also serves as a recreational magnet for fishing, boating, camping, hiking, and bicycling—though the latter two activities are not as popular as the first three. But, again, the springtime flourish can be dazzling.

THE ROUTE

From the starting point, the nearly level trail (an unpaved service road) wraps around the shoreline of the lake. The vegetation on the slopes is primarily of the coastal sage scrub variety, which goes almost completely dormant in drought. The plants pack their growth and reproductive phases into the space of a few weeks or months, depending on how much rain falls. By March, wildflowers such as paintbrush, wild hyacinth, monkey flower, lupine, and owl's clover splash the hillsides with highlights of every hue.

Continue for just 0.8 mile to a point on the trail overlooking Half Moon Cove. Notice the broad saddle in the ridge to your right (north). Leave the trail at that point and climb up about 50 yards to that saddle, where a gorgeous vista opens to the northeast. You look down upon the table-flat floodplain of the San Diego River, and in the distance spot rock-ribbed El Cajon Mountain, whose sheer south face is known as El Capitan in these parts due to its resemblance to El Capitan in Yosemite National Park. Retrace your steps, keeping this route to its intended 1.6-mile, round-trip stroll (plus the little segue to the saddle vista).

Or, you can continue on toward Lake Jennings's rustic campground on the north shore, where paved Bass Drive resumes; that would turn this route into a 2.6-mile outing.

If you don't mind sharing the road with typically slow-moving vehicles, another option would be to circle the lake using Bass Drive—4.6 miles for that entire loop.

TO THE TRAILHEAD
GPS Coordinates: N32° 51.657000'   W116° 53.113382'

Exit I-8 at Lake Jennings Park Road, just east of El Cajon. Go north for about 0.3 mile and turn right onto Harritt Road, following the signs to Lake Jennings. Once past the park entrance, stay right, pay the small day-use fee at the bait shop, and continue driving on the winding, paved Bass Drive along the lake's south and east shorelines. After nearly 2 miles, you reach a parking lot where the paved road ends and a hikers' unpaved trail begins.

46 Father Junipero Serra Trail

Trailhead Location: Between San Diego and Santee

Trail Use: Hiking, biking, dog walking, running, skating, night hiking

Distance & Configuration: 4-mile out-and-back

Elevation Range: 200 feet at the start to 300 feet

Facilities: Water and restrooms at Mission Trails Regional Park Visitor Center and at Old Mission Dam

Highlights: Coastal San Diego County's deepest river gorge

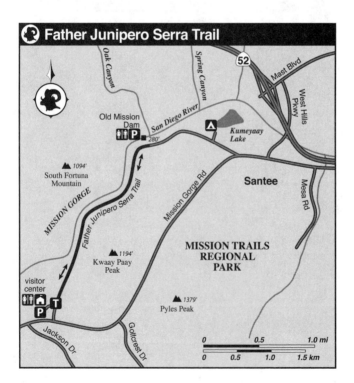

DESCRIPTION

Mission Gorge is arguably the most spectacular topographical feature in the city of San Diego. On both sides of the gorge, walls rise several hundred feet at a nearly 45-degree pitch. From a geological perspective, the gorge was carved out by the "mighty" San Diego River—mighty during Pleistocene times, anyway. The water kept eroding its way through a rising block of tough igneous rock for millions of years. In today's rather dry geologic epoch, there's not as much waterborne excavation going on at the bottom of the gorge, but San Diego's own "old man river" still keeps flowing, mostly lazily, around water-polished granitic rocks and over the roots of gnarled live oaks and rangy sycamores.

THE ROUTE

A single multiuse route threads along the bottom of Mission Gorge today. Actually a paved road called Father Junipero Serra Trail, this route was originally the main, two-lane Mission Gorge Road that connected San Diego's easternmost neighborhoods to Santee. Into the 1960s and '70s, the road still carried secondary car and truck traffic, even after the construction of the four- to six-lane segment of new Mission Gorge Road that bypasses the gorge. Fast-moving semitrucks and recreational cyclists and hikers didn't mix well.

Finally, in the mid-1990s, automotive traffic was nearly eliminated on Father Junipero Serra Trail, and self-propelled travelers at last could feel welcome to use it as a recreational pathway.

The current configuration of Father Junipero Serra Trail is twofold. It features a single, speed-bump-studded, eastbound lane that is open during daylight hours for slow-moving automobiles, and it also offers a wide, separate, parallel path for travelers going either direction by foot, bike, or skates. Dog walking is a popular activity as well.

Plentiful free parking is available at either end of the gorge: at the Old Mission Dam historic site off Mission Gorge Road on Santee's west side and at the Mission Trails Regional Park Visitor Center, just east of the Mission Gorge Road and Jackson Drive intersection. Park near the intersection if you want to include a jaunt to the visitor center before or after your hike. Admission is free, and you'll enjoy interpretive displays and commanding views of the gorge.

At the Old Mission Dam side of the trail, you can walk a short distance down to the remnant dam, built in 1816 by Native American labor secured by the San Diego Mission. The dam, tiny by today's standards, and a 6-mile-long flume facilitated the transfer of water from Mission Gorge to the fertile fields of Mission Valley.

The gently rising and falling 2-mile stretch of paved trail in between the visitor center and the Old Mission Dam offers continual vistas of the

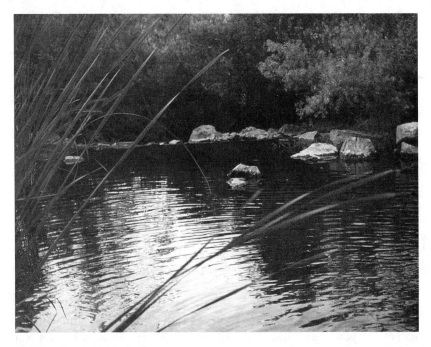

San Diego River inside Mission Gorge

dramatically soaring walls of the gorge. In a couple of spots, you can take side paths down to the bottom of the gorge, where the San Diego River slides gently through the cottonwoods and around boulders fallen from the walls of the gorge. Here and there, especially high on the east side, the gorge's granitic bones form an exoskeleton that attracts technical rock climbers from around the region.

While on the paved pathway, keep an eye out for other travelers—from bicyclists zipping around at high speed to kids and pets darting randomly. Also, use caution when exploring any of the side paths so as to avoid any unpleasant encounters with rattlesnakes.

TO THE TRAILHEAD
GPS Coordinates: N32° 49.183023'   W117° 3.382437'
The main trailhead, at Mission Trails Regional Park's visitor center, lies just north of Mission Gorge Road, one long block east of Jackson Drive (approximately 4 miles north and east of the Mission Gorge Road exit at I-8, and approximately 5 miles west of Santee's city center).

47 Oak Canyon

Trailhead Location: Mission Gorge, west of Santee

Trail Use: Hiking, dog walking

Distance & Configuration: 3-mile out-and-back

Elevation Range: 280 feet near the start to 590 feet

Facilities: Water and portable toilets at the trailhead

Highlights: A small stream with mini-waterfalls; extravagant springtime vegetation

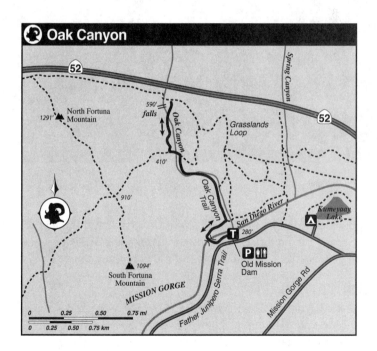

DESCRIPTION

Oak Canyon, a sycamore- and oak-lined ravine that winds north from Mission Gorge's Old Mission Dam, is a perfect place to celebrate the return of spring in San Diego. Heavy rains revive the canyon's intermittent stream and transform the hillside vegetation from dormant brown to

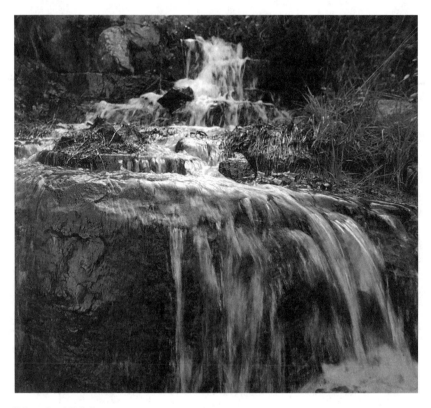

Winter flood, Oak Canyon

festive green. By March, annual wildflowers pop up amid the tender new blades of grass, blooming ceanothus (wild lilac) color the slopes, and the sweet-pungent smell of sage floats on the warm breezes.

THE ROUTE

From the Old Mission Dam parking area, walk west down the wide, smooth path going past various interpretive exhibits and the Old Mission Dam. The dam was built 1807–1816 under the direction of the San Diego Mission and was considered a major engineering feat of its day. A 6-mile-long flume carried water from the dam to the mission at the east end of Mission Valley.

Beyond the exhibits, you cross the often-turbid waters of the San Diego River by way of an iron footbridge. The trail then traverses a sandy stretch of river floodplain and bends right (east) to climb a hillside. After about 100 yards, stay left and descend to the bottom of a shallow ravine—Oak Canyon. In the next 1.2 miles, you'll wend your way upstream along the banks of the trickling creek, passing small cascades and rock-bound pools (in season, of course). Small kids may need a hand in places, and they should be kept well away from the sheer drops where the stream has carved deep into the bedrock. Everyone will enjoy cottontail rabbits scampering through the brush. With some luck, you might flush a covey of quail. Coyotes patrol these spaces, but unless the hour is either very early or very late, you'll likely see no more than tracks and scat.

Avoid any trails that branch right, away from the canyon bottom. After a total of 1.2 miles, the path intersects a dirt access road to power lines. Turn left, follow the road about 100 yards, and go right on a path that continues up Oak Canyon. About 0.3 mile farther, you'll come to a picturesque mini-chasm of water-polished rock with a deep, narrow pool. You could walk farther, but this route ends here, as SR 52 passes over the canyon just ahead on twin high bridges, and off-limits Marine Corps property lies beyond.

TO THE TRAILHEAD
GPS Coordinates: N32° 50.361543'   W117° 2.570822'
From Mission Gorge Road on Santee's west side, drive 0.7 mile west on Father Junipero Serra Trail to the Old Mission Dam parking lot on the right. If this lot is full, there is plenty of overflow parking available on the road shoulder outside.

48 Cowles Mountain

Trailhead Location: San Diego's San Carlos neighborhood, on the city's east side

Trail Use: Hiking, dog walking, running

Distance & Configuration: 3-mile out-and-back

Elevation Range: 658 feet at the trailhead to 1,591 feet at the top

Facilities: Water and restrooms at the trailhead; snack shop and convenience store across the street

Highlights: Simply the most comprehensive vista any peak in San Diego can offer

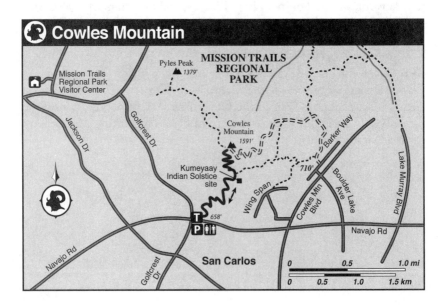

DESCRIPTION

For good reason, this switchback trail is the most heavily trafficked hiking route in all of San Diego County. The route ascends the sunny south side of Cowles Mountain to the summit—the highest point within San Diego's city limits. Because of the low-growing vegetation, you and your fellow hikers will enjoy unobstructed views nearly the entire way up. At first, nearby features such as Lake Murray command your attention. Then far-off locales—Mexico, downtown San Diego, and the Pacific Ocean—come into view.

The trail was cut on mostly decomposed granite, so it is quite susceptible to erosion wherever the slope gets steep. Please don't shortcut the switchbacks, tempting as it may be on the way up or down, as this aggravates the erosion problem. Wear sturdy shoes, as jutting rocks and wicked little ruts sometimes punctuate the trail surface. Also, consider not doing this climb when the weather is hot and sunny. It's easy to become dehydrated and woozy, and you'll need all of your faculties to negotiate the rough patches on the way down. Carry along plenty of drinking water, of course.

THE ROUTE

From the trailhead, make your way up the zigzagging and occasionally heavily eroded trail, which climbs relentlessly through low-growing sage scrub and chaparral. By 0.7 mile, you're passing scattered outcrops of rounded granitic rock, which add to the aesthetic pleasure of the widening panorama. At a spot 0.9 mile beyond your starting point, the main trail bends sharply left.

At that bend, an obscure path continues straight ahead about 50 yards to a flat spot on the mountain's south shoulder. This optional side trip is worth exploring. Precisely on that flat spot, there once existed a circular array of stones crossed by an arrow-configuration of rocks pointing to where the winter solstice sun rises every December 20 or 21. This Kumeyaay (Native American) solstice site is a place where hikers converge at dawn on the appropriate date to view the rising sun's upper rim momentarily split in two pieces by a distant rock pillar.

Back on the main trail, a little farther upslope, at 1 mile from the start, a through-trail branches right, heading eastward toward Barker Way at the mountain's east base. Stay left and continue up the mountainside on the series of long switchback segments leading to the rocky summit of the mountain. A concrete monument marks the high point, and two large interpretive panels stand nearby, with the names and directions of major features visible along the horizon.

A blocky building bristling with microwave dishes obstructs the northward view somewhat, but otherwise the panorama is complete. With binoculars and a street map, you may be lulled into spending a lot of time identifying features on the urban landscape. In the rift between the coastal

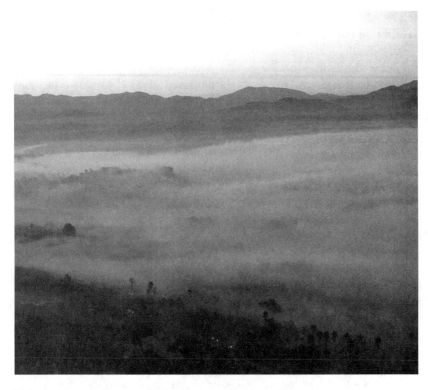

Early morning marine layer over San Diego, as seen from Cowles Mountain

terrace to the west, there's a good view of Mission Valley and the tangle of freeways that pass over and through it. Southwest, the high-rise buildings of downtown San Diego stand against Point Loma, Coronado, and San Diego Bay. Lake Murray shimmers to the south. The chain of Santee Lakes contrasts darkly with pale hills to the north. In all directions, you look down on the abodes of many of the more than 4 million people who live within a 35-mile radius of where you stand.

On clear winter days, the view expands to include most of the higher peaks of San Diego County. Southward into Baja, you can see the flat-topped Table Mountain beyond Tijuana and the Coronado Islands offshore. During absolutely crystalline weather, look for the profiles of Santa Catalina and San Clemente islands, to the northwest and west respectively.

After you've gaped sufficiently at the surrounding landscape, or perhaps finished your trailside snack or lunch, turn around and return exactly as you came. But be especially cautious on the way down. Remember those steep and eroded sections of trail that you covered on the way up? Observe such rough areas and descend accordingly. As noted in the Introduction, this is a very popular trail but arguably presents the most challenging descent among all 50 routes in this book.

TO THE TRAILHEAD

GPS Coordinates: N32° 48.291121'   W117° 2.244902'

Exit I-8 at College Avenue, and go north for 1 mile. Turn right onto Navajo Road, and continue 2 miles east to the Cowles Mountain Trailhead on the northeast corner of Navajo Road and Golfcrest Drive.

49 Lake Murray

Trailhead Location: La Mesa, just east of San Diego

Trail Use: Hiking, dog walking, running, biking, skating, night hiking

Distance & Configuration: 6-mile out-and-back

Elevation Range: About 550 feet throughout

Facilities: Water, restrooms, and small concession stand at the start; pit toilets along the route; water at a drinking fountain next to some baseball fields at Lake Murray Community Park on the north shore

Highlights: Fresh breezes and sparkling lake views all along the route; superb bird-watching opportunities

DESCRIPTION

Lake Murray is eastern San Diego's most pleasant and most popular place to gulp some fresh air just about any time of year. Earlier or later on most days, hundreds of runners, speed walkers, skaters, and cyclists dodge each other on the lake's perimeter service road (closed to autos) that extends along about four-fifths of the lake's shoreline. Thus, the road's end, about 3 miles out from the start, makes this route an out-and-back rather than a pleasing lake loop.

Lake Murray is also considered to be one of the five best bird-watching locales in San Diego County. Be sure to bring binoculars to visually capture the lake's mix of aquatic fowl (ducks, coots, white pelicans, great blue herons, and much more) and also the freewheeling large birds (hawks, ravens, and vultures) in the sky overhead.

THE ROUTE

From the easternmost parking area beyond the lake entrance, start your walk at the perimeter road, which is gated to block vehicles. Eucalyptus and jacaranda trees spread shade over the road along the way, but mostly this route is open to the warm sun; thus hikers and runners much prefer the early morning and late afternoon hours. (A contingent of early risers from the adjacent neighborhood often walks the lake route as early as 5 a.m.)

After swinging around four fingerlike arms of the lake, the publicly accessible part of the road comes to an end at a formidable fence just shy of the west abutment of the Lake Murray Dam. There's no passage across

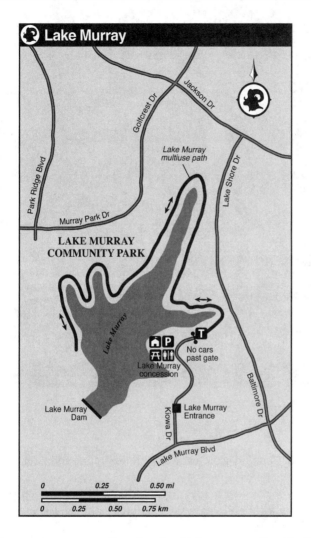

Lake Murray

Golfcrest Dr

Jackson Dr

Lake Murray
multiuse path

Park Ridge Blvd

Lake Shore Dr

Murray Park Dr

LAKE MURRAY
COMMUNITY PARK

Lake Murray

No cars
past gate

Lake Murray
concession

Lake Murray
Dam

Kiowa Dr

Lake Murray
Entrance

Baltimore Dr

Lake Murray Blvd

| 0 | 0.25 | 0.50 mi |
| 0 | 0.25 | 0.50 | 0.75 km |

the narrow concrete dam ahead, which was completed in 1918, so you must turn back and return from there.

You'll likely enjoy this far-end section of the perimeter road best. A wild, rocky, scruffy hillside rises to the west, housing a cohort of coyotes, whose howls announce their presence after dark. To the east spreads the sometimes glassy, sometimes wind-rippled surface of the lake, flecked with rowboats and small fishing craft.

On your way back from the turnaround point, you may consider following any of several paralleling trails that diverge from and later return to

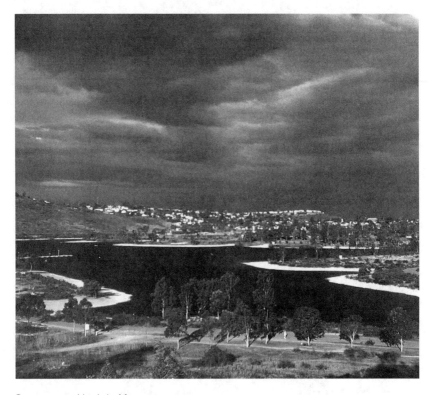

Storm approaching Lake Murray

the paved main road. You will see them along the shoreline and along the slopes above the perimeter road.

Another activity to consider here is night hiking. You can park outside the entrance gate, walk in, and enjoy the shadowy sights and nocturnal sounds along the lakeshore.

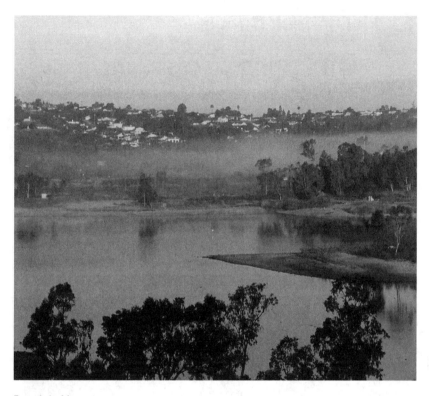

Foggy Lake Murray

TO THE TRAILHEAD

GPS Coordinates: N32° 47.100420'   W117° 2.495699'

From I-8 in La Mesa, take the Lake Murray Boulevard exit. Drive 0.5 mile north to Kiowa Drive, and turn left. Kiowa dead-ends at the Lake Murray gate, which is open during daylight hours. Parking is free in several lots inside.

50 Hollenbeck Canyon

Trailhead Location: East of Jamul in southern San Diego County

Trail Use: Hiking, dog walking, running, mountain biking, horseback riding

Distance & Configuration: 4-mile out-and-back

Elevation Range: 700–1,100 feet

Facilities: None at the trailhead; all are in Jamul, 4 miles west

Highlights: Stunning springtime-green vegetation and wildflowers

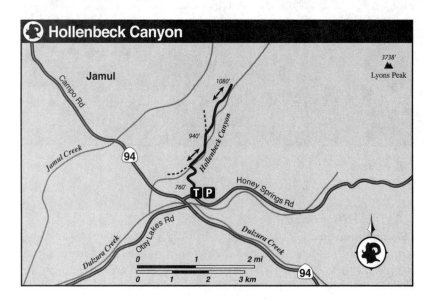

DESCRIPTION

Formerly part of a working ranch, Hollenbeck Canyon is now a California Department of Fish and Game wildlife area. It is open to all types of nonmotorized travel, plus a bit of seasonal bird hunting. Like many low-elevation inland locales in San Diego County, Hollenbeck Canyon has a Jekyll-and-Hyde personality, sun-blasted and desolate for the most part in summer and gloriously green—almost lush—in the winter and early spring. This dichotomy is due purely to the prevailing winter-wet, summer-dry climate. Down along the canyon bottom itself, however, water (either on the surface or underground during the dry seasons) nourishes shade-giving trees. And the shrubby and grassy hillside vegetation that goes dormant during drought comes alive with frenzied growth in the weeks following the winter rains. For this reason, January–April is typically the best time to hike here.

THE ROUTE

From the trailhead parking area, a 0.3-mile passage across an often-parched, treeless meadow hardly prepares you for the idyllic scene soon to come. You pass a yellow-topped post marking the route of the historic California Riding and Hiking Trail and descend gently into shallow Hollenbeck Canyon. At this point, the canyon is lined by an agreeable collection of massive coast live oaks and leafy California sycamores. One of the first oaks in sight is a grizzled, misshapen specimen that not only has survived past fires but that also soars some 50 feet into the sky. The trail soon curves left to cross the canyon's seasonal stream and joins a dirt road. Stay right—and remember this juncture on your way back when you will be tracing this same route backward.

Onward, you go alongside a thin green strip of willow trees, mule fat shrubs, and other riparian vegetation, with a stray Engelmann oak or two joining the coast live oaks and sycamores. The slopes of the canyon, clothed in a veneer of sage scrub vegetation, gradually close in tighter. From this vantage, no sign of civilization save the road you walk upon is apparent. The wind whispers in fluttering leaves.

At 1.3 miles from the start, a side path goes left about 50 yards to the foundation remains of a cabin. Stay on the main route, and soon afterward, a side trail diverges to the right from the wider path that climbs upward along a broad ridge. Take the more interesting of the two—the path to the right. It threads the eroded west wall of the narrowing gorge ahead. At 2 miles total, a yellow sign identifies the property line of the wildlife area you are in. At that spot, there's a vertiginous view into the narrows of Hollenbeck Canyon, where floodwaters tumbling down from upstream Lyons Valley have cut a nearly vertical trench in the bedrock. Off in the distance, eastward, soars the rocky summit of Lyons Peak.

Here, you've reached the end of the line; turn around and retrace the same 2 miles back to the trailhead, staying left at each junction.

TO THE TRAILHEAD

GPS Coordinates: N32° 40.242898'   W116° 49.389961'

From San Diego, take SR 94 east. Continue beyond where the freeway ends, and at the third traffic light (Campo Road), turn right to remain on SR 94. Continue 5 miles to the rural community of Jamul, and go an additional 4 miles on SR 94 to Honey Springs Road, on the left. Make a left, go 0.1 mile, and enter the large parking lot to the left, which serves as the Hollenbeck Canyon Trailhead and equestrian staging area.

INDEX

A

Afoot & Afield San Diego County (Wilderness Press), 1
Alcazar Gardens, 118
animal hazards, 7–8
Armada Terrace, 94, 95
Arroyo Canyon, 110
Asian district, 132

B

B Street Pier, 126
Backesto Building, 131
backpacks, 5–6
Balboa Park, 67, 115
Balboa Park's Central Mesa, 116–118
Balboa Park's East Side, 119–121
Balboa Park's West Mesa, 112–115
Bankers Hill, 108–111
Barnett Ranch Preserve, 53–55
Batiquitos Lagoon, 15–16
Bayside Trail, 90–92
Bayside Walk, 86, 87
Bennington Memorial Oak Grove, 121
Bernardo Mountain, 41–43
Bird Park, 120
bird-watching, best hikes for, x

Bishop's Day School, 109
Black's Beach, 77
Blue Sky Ecological Reserve, 64–65
Boardwalk, the, 24
Bonita, 139
book, using this, 4–9
Botanical Building, Balboa Park, 117
Broadway Pier, 126–127
butterflies, 14

C

Cabrillo Freeway, 118
Cabrillo National Monument, 91, 92
Cave Store, the, 79
cell phones, 7
Central Mesa, Balboa Park, 116–118
children, best hikes for small, xi
Chula Vista, 141
Circling Sail Bay, 86–89
Clevenger Canyon, 50
Coast to Crest Trail, 23–24
Coast Walk, 78–80
Coastal & Central San Diego
   See also specific hike
   featured hikes, 68–135
   map, 66
   regional overview, 4, 67

C (*continued*)

Coastal North County
    See also specific hike
    featured hikes, 12–29
    map, 10
    regional overview, 4, 11
Cobbleback Peak, 56
Congo River Fishing Village, 48
Coronado Beach, 133–135
Cowles Mountain, 162–165

D

Daley Ranch preserve, 44
Dana Landing, 86, 88
D.A.R. (Daughters of the American
    Revolution) Trail, 27
Del, the, 134
Del Dios Gorge, 38–40
Del Mar Crest & Beach, 25–29
Discovery Lake, 33, 34
Discovery Park, 142
Dog Beach, 134
dog walking, best hikes for, x
Double Peak, 32–34

E

East County
    See also specific hike
    featured hikes, 150–172
    map, 148
    regional overview, 4, 149
El Cajon Mountain, 154
elevation, selecting hikes by, 4–5
Elfin Forest Recreational Reserve, 35–37
Embarcadero, the, 125–128
Embarcadero Marine Park, 128
equipment, suggested hiking, 5–7
Escondido Creek, 36
eucalyptus trees, 13–14

F

Father Junipero Serra Trail, 156–158
Felicita Creek, 42–43
First San Diego River Improvement
    Project, 103
Florida Canyon, Balboa Park, 120–121

G

Gaslamp Quarter, 129–132
geology, selecting hikes by, 4–5
Gill, Irving, 109, 110

H

Harbor Island, 99–101
hikes
    See also specific hike
    Coastal & Central San Diego, 68–135
    Coastal North County, 12–29
    East County, 150–172
    Inland North County, 30–65
    selecting, 4–5
    South County, 136–147
    very best short, x–xi
hiking
    elevation and, 2
    'leave no trace,' 8
    precautions, 5–8
    safety, 5–8
Hollenbeck Canyon, 170–172
Horton Plaza fountain, 131, 132
Hosp Grove, 12–14
Hotel del Coronado, xii, 134, 135
Hubbell, James, 97

I

Imperial Beach, 145–147
Inland North County
    See also specific hike
    featured hikes, 32–65
    map, 30

regional overview, 4, 31
Iron Mountain, 59–61
Italy, Little, 111

J

Jack Creek Meadow, 44–46
Japanese Friendship Garden, 118

K

Keating Building, 131
Kellogg Park, 75, 76
Kumeyaay Promontory, 152
Kumeyaay solstice site, 163

L

La Jolla, 81
La Jolla Caves, 78, 79
La Jolla Shores, 75–77
La Playa & Point Loma, 93–95
Lake Hodges, 36, 37, 42, 43
Lake Hodges Dam, 38, 39, 40
Lake Jennings, 153–155
Lake Murray, 163, 164, 166–169
Lake Poway Loop, 62–63
Lake Poway Recreation Area, 65
legend, map, 9
lemonade berry bushes, 142
lions, mountain, 8
Little Italy neighborhood, 111
Los Penasquitos Canyon, 72–74
Louis Bank of Commerce building, 131
Louis Stelzer County Park, 150–152
Lower Otay County Park, 143–144

M

maps
    See also specific hike
    Coastal & Central San Diego, 66
    Coastal North County, 10
    East County, 148
    Inland North County, 30
    legend, 9
    San Diego, vi
    South County, 136
Marian Bear Memorial Park, 84–85
Maritime Museum of San Diego,
    125–126
Marston House, 115
MiraCosta College, 21, 22
Mission Bay Park, 67
Mission Beach, 86
Mission Gorge, 157–158
Mission Valley, 157
Mission Valley San Diego River Trail,
    102–104
monarch butterflies, 14
Morley Field dog park, 120
mountain lions, 8
Mountain of Moonlit Rocks, 56
Multiple Species Conservation Program,
    54
Museum of Man's California Tower, 115,
    118

N

Navy Pier, 127

O

Oak Canyon, 159–161
Ocean Beach, 104
Ocean Front Walk, 86
Old Mission Dam, 157, 159, 160
Old Point Loma Lighthouse,
    91–92
Olivenhain Dam & Reservoir,
    36, 37
Organ Pavilion, 118
Otay Mountain, 144

P

Pacific Flyway, 146
Pacific International Exposition site,
    116–117
Pacific Portal (sculpture), 97
Panama-California Exposition site,
    116–117
Pearl of the Pacific (sculpture), 97
plants, hazardous, 7
Plaza de Panama, 117, 118
Point Loma, 90–91, 93–95
poison oak, 7
Powerhouse Park, 27
Prospect Street, 80

R

raingear, 6
Ramona Reservoir Dam, 65
Ramona Valley, 57
rattlesnakes, 7
Redwood Circle, 115
Rice Canyon, 141–142
Ridgetop Picnic Area, 37
Riviera Shores, 88
Rose Canyon Open Space, 85
Royal Food Mart, 111
running, best hikes for, x–xi

S

safe hiking tips, 5–8
Sail Bay, 86–89
San Clemente Canyon, 85
San Diego
    See also specific region
    introduction and overview, 1–3
    overview map, vi
    regional designations, 4–5
San Diego City Hall building, old, 131
San Diego Natural History Museum, 117
San Diego River, 104, 157, 158, 160
San Diego Zoo, 122–124
San Diego Zoo Safari Park, 47–49, 122
San Dieguito Lagoon, 23–24
San Dieguito River, 39
San Dieguito River Park, 41, 50
San Elijo Hills housing development, 33
San Elijo Lagoon, 20–22
San Elijo State Beach, 19
San Miguel Mountain, 139
San Pasqual Trails South, 50–52
Santa Rosa Island, 68
Santee Lakes, 164
Scripps Park, 80
Scripps Pier, 76
Seagrove Park, 27
Seaport Village, 128
Self-Realization Fellowship retreat,
    17–18
Sessions, Kate, 115
Shelter Island, 96–98
small children, best hikes for, xi
Soledad Mountain, 81–83
South County
    See also specific hike
    featured hikes, 136–147
    map, 136
    regional overview, 4, 137
Southwestern College, 142
springtime wildflowers, best hikes for, xi
Star of India ship, 125–126
Stelzer Park, 151, 152
Sunny Jim Cave, 79
Swami's Beach, 17–19
Sweetwater Trail, 138–140
Switzer Canyon, 120
symbols, map, 9

T

Table Mountain, 164
Tecolote Canyon, 105–107
Tecolote Canyon Natural Park, 106
Tecolote Community Park, 107
temperatures in San Diego area, 2
ticks, 7
Tijuana River Estuary, 146
Tom Ham's Lighthouse
    Restaurant, 101
Torrey Pines City Beach, 77
Torrey Pines Glider Port, 71
Torrey Pines State Reserve, 26, 68–71
Trees for Health Garden, 115
Tuna Harbor Park, 127–128
Tunaman's Memorial (sculpture), 97

U

Urban Trees (sculpture), 125, 127
US Grant Hotel, 131

V

very best short hikes, x–xi
vistas, best hikes for, xi
Volcan Mountain, 23

W

water, 5, 7
Waterman, Waldo, 108
weather in San Diego area, 2
West Mesa, Balboa Park, 112–115
Wildcat Canyon, 151, 152
wildflowers, best hikes for, xi
wildlife-watching, best hikes for, x
William Heath Davis House, 131
Wings of the World aviary, 47
Woodson Mountain, 56–58

Y

Yogananda, Paramahansa, 17
Yokohama Friendship Bell (sculpture), 97

About the Author

Jerry Schad
1949–2011

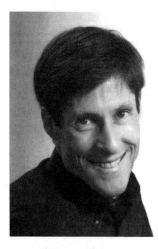

photographed by eabrownstudio.com

The author's several careers encompassed interests ranging from astronomy and teaching to photography and writing. Jerry Schad held bachelor's and master's degrees in astronomy, taught physical science and astronomy at San Diego Mesa College, and chaired the Mesa College Physical Sciences Department.

Schad was the author of 15 books, including a college-level textbook for introductory physical science courses and the top-selling *Afoot & Afield* series of hiking guidebooks that cover nearly all of Southern California. He became interested in astronomy at age 12, took up astronomical photography a few years later, and had some 1,500 astronomical photographs published in media around the world.

Schad's outdoor column, "Roam-O-Rama," was published weekly in the *San Diego Reader* 1993–2011, and his *San Diego Reader* blog, "Outdoor San Diego," kept San Diegans up-to-date on a variety of natural events in the sky and on earth.

At one time, Schad ran a 100-mile trail race across the Sierra Nevada in 24 hours. He also bicycled 352 miles from San Jose to the outskirts of Los Angeles in even less time.

In the last year of his life, Schad enjoyed spending time with his wife, Peg Reiter, as they walked, hiked, traveled, and enjoyed time in their high-rise residential tower in downtown San Diego.

In the months preceding his death at age 61 from kidney cancer, Schad worked tirelessly and with courageous joy and spirit to complete the final stages of this book.

Other Books by Jerry Schad from Wilderness Press

Afoot & Afield Orange County

In 87 hikes in the parks, preserves, designated open spaces, and public lands surrounding Orange County's densely populated coastal plain, this book provides fresh inspiration for trips along the coast from Huntington Beach to San Clemente, in the rugged Santa Ana Mountains, and through the foothills from Anaheim to the Santa Rosa Plateau Ecological Reserve.

ISBN 978-0-89997-397-5

Afoot & Afield Los Angeles County

This guide covers all the best LA adventures, from strolling along at Malibu Lagoon State Beach to trekking up a mountain on Catalina Island. Choose from 200 trips to explore the City of Angels' own backyard, traveling through a variety of climate zones and revealing a remarkably diverse array of plant and animal life.

ISBN 978-0-89997-499-6

Afoot & Afield San Diego County

This fourth edition of San Diego County's classic hiking guidebook features 250 trips, ranging from short, self-guiding nature trails to challenging peak climbs and canyon treks. The book encompasses almost all public—and a few private—lands within San Diego County, including Anza-Borrego Desert State Park, Cleveland National Forest, the Cuyamaca Mountains, and numerous county and city parks.

ISBN 978-0-89997-428-6

101 Hikes in Southern California

This book proves there's more to SoCal than theme parks and strip malls. From the San Gabriel Mountains to the Anza-Borrego Desert and everywhere in between, this guide offers an incredible selection of exciting trips covering scores of hidden places just beyond the urban horizon.

ISBN 978-0-89997-351-7

Top Trails Los Angeles

This highly visual guide to 48 of the Southland's best trails in the greater LA metro area, from Malibu to the Hollywood Hills, San Jacinto Peak to the San Fernando Valley, includes trail feature tables, don't-get-lost milestones, maps for every trip, and more.

ISBN 978-0-89997-627-3

Trail Runner's Guide: San Diego

A comprehensive guide to running the myriad trails of sun-soaked San Diego, from the beach at La Jolla to the summit of Palomar Mountain, includes climate and topography tips, maps, photographs, and more. Runners and hikers alike will appreciate the detailed descriptions of 50 exhilarating routes.

ISBN 978-0-89997-308-1

For ordering information, contact your local
bookseller or Wilderness Press.
www.wildernesspress.com